# SEXTUPLETS

# SEXTUPLETS
## Study of a sibling group

*Linda Root Fortini and Laura Mori*

Translated from Italian by Diana Sears
Originally published as
*Fratelli e sorelle coetanei—studio su una gemellarità plurima*

## KARNAC

First published in 2010 by
Karnac Books Ltd
118 Finchley Road
London NW3 5HT

British Library Cataloguing in Publication Data

A C.I.P. for this book is available from the British Library

ISBN-13: 978-1-85575-564-2

Typeset by Vikatan Publishing Solutions (P) Ltd., Chennai, India


www.karnacbooks.com

# CONTENTS

*ACKNOWLEDGEMENTS*                                       vii

*FOREWORD*                                                ix

*PREFACE*
Gina Ferrara Mori and Franco Mori                         xv

*INTRODUCTION*                                           xxi

*CHAPTER ONE*
Research methods and structure                             1

*CHAPTER TWO*
Infancy and childhood as seen through *infant observation*   7

*CHAPTER THREE*
Psychodynamic profiles of the individual sextuplets       39

*CHAPTER FOUR*
Being in six                                              73

*CHAPTER FIVE*
Follow-up fifteen years later             93

*CLOSING COMMENTS*             129

*REFERENCES*             133

*INDEX*             139

# *ACKNOWLEDGEMENTS*

We wish to express our gratitude to the mother and the entire family of the sextuplets for their collaboration in the realization of this research study. We have respected as much as possible the personal privacy of each individual family member in our preparation of this publication.

We also wish to thank our colleagues, friends and relatives whose ideas and thoughts helped us in our investigations on the main themes of the book and in the organization of the material, text revisions, and elaboration of the tables, graphs and figures.

# FOREWORD

The topic of this book is immensely interesting. Linda Fortini had a unique opportunity to study a family of sextuplets. And she chose a unique method—one based on the psychoanalytic observation of infants and mothers which has not been used with a family of this kind. This book is a record of the development of the family in the first two years, but not only that; in addition there is a quite complex follow-up study of the children into early adulthood using material from interviews and psychological testing. Linda's aim, together with the assistance of her colleague, Laura Mori, was to explore possible correlations between early infantile experience and later personality development.

The key method is that of psychoanalytic infant observation established by Esther Bick (1964) in the 1950s, and this study is a significant and original addition to the literature on that method of observation. At first the method was to sensitise trainee child psychotherapists and psychoanalysts to their specific field of study—the relatedness between baby and mother (Briggs 2002). However, from early on psychoanalytic infant observation began to produce original research results (Bick 1968), and this has been a growing activity (Reid et al ** 19**, Rustin, et al 19**). The method has been standardised and has its place beside, and in parallel with, other more experimental methods of investigating mother-infant psychology. It is a naturalistic method in which the observer goes into the normal environment of the subjects of the study; it is a kind of anthropological fieldwork, with both the limitations and advantages of such a method.

Whereas this method has previously been used to investigate apparently normal families and the development of ordinary children, in this study the family is quite extraordinary. This is not just a large family. This is an overwhelming family—albeit without an intention to deprive. Even in ordinary large families, each successive baby does have a more or less exclusive relationship with maternal care, for a period immediately after birth. In this family none of the children ever get that exclusivity.

Everyone knows the stress on the family when a new baby arrives. However, the arrival of six new babies all at once is hard to imagine. One gets the impression of just what an undertaking it is. Two parents are simply not enough, and the extended family has to be called in as recruits, as well as neighbours and more official helpers. As these observations show the overwhelming clamour of neediness from six babies appears to dominate the family, and one's anxiety on behalf of the needy children makes it difficult to reflect on the impact this makes on the reader. He gapes with admiration and shock at what the impact must have been like for the children themselves, who knew nothing else, and on the rest of the family who, to be realistic, also knew nothing else like it.

The family and its helpers were turned into a dedicated team of carers, but one remains concerned at what level of care could have been provided. This powerful impact of concern no doubt reflects the flood of concern within the family itself. That impact rubs off on the observer and ultimately the reader. In fact, in this method a direct transfer of feelings to the observer inevitably occurs, and thus enables a deeper reflection in terms of personal experiencing through a consideration of the observer's experience. This quality of being overwhelmed by urgent physical needs is vivid in the observer, but it had no doubt been transferred in turn from the experience of the newborn baby at birth. The observer reflects the unease such that the reader 'reads' those feelings as well as the words.

Any baby is confronted with the challenges of a life separate in body and mind, and assaulted by completely new sensations and mental proto-experiences. At birth a baby's experience must include that helplessness with the unfamiliarity of its own experiences, and its lack of comprehension of how to satisfy itself. That, after all, is why mothers exist; a baby born into incomprehension and helplessness is in Winnicott's terms only a part of a whole system, a system that consists of mother and baby together as the unit. Maternal care has not only to give bodily satisfaction in the right way at the right time, it must also do so in a way that addresses the experiences of incomprehension and helplessness. This family had to endure the impact six-fold, throughout an almost indefinite period into the future.

In baby care, the management of psychic functioning is, we know, just as important as the physical satisfaction and care. This study rightly homes in on this. It picks up on the problem of the psychic space that is available for these experiences, and the observations note very intensely the uncomfortable sense of inadequate space. The children crowd each other, and they jostle each other, in ways which seem to express that struggle to find a personal space or territory. It makes the mother think about what it must have been like inside the womb.

The focus on space makes one think of Esther Bick's results from the original use of this method. She too found herself focusing down on the experience of space—and its boundaries. Working of course mostly with families with one newborn, it became apparent that skin contact was an essential pre-requisite for developing a sense of completeness. The physical skin represents, and is felt actually to *be*, the ego boundary. It needs constant stimulus at the outset of life to establish that identity of the self. Swaddling, cuddling and rocking all give that foundational skin stimulus which primes the new little person to feel the boundaries of his space, and thus his sense of self. By feeling bounded by the world, the infant can come to experience the necessary boundary *in* itself, that makes it feel complete. Moreover, Bick observed that where there is a deficient degree of skin contact and stimulation, the infant resorts to other substitute methods of holding itself together. These 'second-skin' phenomena, might be a precocious holding on to a light source, or a noise, or making repetitive noises, or keeping its muscle tone rigid to 'hold' himself. The present observations on this jostling and physical play may represent the possibility of appeasing the need for bodily

contact and comfort with others. That is to say, they help each other
to sense their ego-boundaries through skin sensation of each other
in their jostling. How much then do these children gain a comfort
from each other? And this reminds one of Pierre Turquet's (1975)
idea about the way that individuals us the 'skin-of-my-neighbour'
to define their own identity in the large group. When the observer,
and the reader, spot the problem of personal space, this may be the
direct transfer to the sensitive observer, which points to the equally
sensitive and profound struggle by the babies to begin the development of self, boundary, and identity.

Given the apparent difficulties, intense from the outset of life, it
is surprising that so many of the babies emerged as normal enough
adults. However, two of them, the middle two, conspicuously did
not achieve a normal development. One of the infants suffered particularly from the lack of exclusivity of maternal care, and the study
shows that he precisely was the one with a slow and inadequate
development, and both mental and emotional deficiencies. Meeting
him again as a young adult he had remained the most dependent on
the family (parents and siblings), had limited social and intellectual
capacities, and had developed a chronic illness in adolescence. Psychological disturbance, it seems, came to be progressively located in
this particular child in contrast to most of the others who seemed to
achieve a freedom to mature normally. This might make us turn to
group dynamic phenomena such as that of 'scapegoating'. Indeed
with an infant observation of so many infants one might need to be
a group therapist as well as a psychoanalyst to fully comprehend
the phenomena on view. In other words did that child grow up as
the emblem of the disturbance that all of them felt? Understood in
group relations terms, that implies an important and unconscious
emotional role was allotted, and accepted, by the child. So could
that unconscious, emotional role, which sacrificed one, enable others to be sufficiently free of disturbance to attain an ordinary enough
personality?

Inevitably, with such an original, logistically difficult and complex study, the observational method was perforce modified. For
instance, after birth the infants were immediately separated from
mother and from each other, by being looked after in the clinical environment of an incubator. This complication prevented infant-mother
observation in the normal setting from being established until the

babies were six months of age. One wonders about the impact on the development of sibling relations after the separation, and whether the observations are a record in part of that early PTSD. Despite such limitations, this is a milestone in the observation method, and later researchers are challenged to repeat this, and perhaps to find a way of investigating these earliest moments of separation.

This research study deserves to be widely read. It is pertinent in our contemporary world where assisted conceptions and multiple births are increasingly frequent. It is also a remarkable use of the psychoanalytic observational method as a planned research tool. Linda and her back-up team have given us a first insight into the turmoil of experience in such contemporary families. And she is to be congratulated on her achievement as much as the family she observed are to be congratulated on rearing som many 'normal' children.

Bob Hinshelwood

Bick, Esther 1964. Notes on infant observation in psychoanalytic training. *International Journal of Psychoanalysis*, 45: 558–566.

Bick, Esther 1968. The experience of the skin in early object relations. *International Journal of Psychoanalysis*, 49: 484–486.

Briggs, Andrew (ed.) 2002. *Surviving Space: Papers on Infant Observation* London: Karnac.

Reid, Sue (ed.) 1997. *Developments in Infant Observation*. London: Routledge.

Miller, Lisa, Rustin, Margaret, Rustin. Michael, and Suttleworth, Judy 1989. *Closely Observed Infants*. London: Duckworth.

Turquet, Pierre 1975. Threats to identity in the large group. In Lionel Kreeger (ed.) *The Large Group*. London: Constable.

# PREFACE

This is a study of an exceptional group of sextuplets who were observed at home on a monthly basis for two-hour visits over a three-year period by Linda Root Fortini, a psychologist who lives and works in Florence, Italy. We remember those meetings more than 20 years ago when we, six participants like the group of sextuplets, discussed the monthly observations. Our group consisted of a paediatrician, a neonatalogist, an auxologist, two psychoanalysts and the author as observer. We all had a common interest in research on child mental development and we followed the traditional methodology of *Infant Observation* established in 1948 at the Tavistock Clinic by Esther Bick, a psychoanalyst.

In each seminar group, also held at monthly intervals, an observation was read and then discussed in depth by the six group members. There was an attempt to give meaning to the various interactions noted between the children and the mother, the children and the observer, and the children and the other people present in the observations. This particular situation might provide insight into other possible events that could occur in a childhood community and in the relationship between such a community and the participating adults, including other involved individuals as well as family members.

Thinking back to those many group discussions we are reminded that this was a completely new experience for all of us. There was a totally free and enriching exchange of ideas, many of which had already matured in our various specialized fields of work.

Uniting our different expertise and varied professional experiences, we were able to comprehend this complex family situation that also involved emotional responses in the seminar members who furnished important support to the observer. Although an expert in *Infant Observation* she, too, was faced with a new experience insofar as the method was being applied to a group of babies rather than the usual mother-child dyad. These observational experiences provide the basis for this book.

We hope that this observational study of the formation of the individual personalities in a group of sextuplets, within the context of a very unusual sibling group and the family itself, will confirm Esther Bick's method as a research tool in the field of infant development. We are aware that this is uncharted territory, but know that we have used valid tools, which, almost to our surprise, we were able to apply usefully and correctly.

After 15 years had elapsed since the completion of the original observations, Linda Root Fortini called in her colleague Laura Mori and together they began a new phase of investigation, renewing the study on the development of the sextuplets by following them from their 18th to their 21st birthday. They followed the study aware of the originality of the project and its conclusions over the lives of the sextuplets documented in this book, which is based principally on the use of observation as a research tool.

Chapter two is dedicated to the elaboration of the most significant observations and relative inferences that arose in the 31 discussions that took place in the first three years of the sextuplets' lives. There is an integration of this information with an overview of the pre-history or *pre-infancy* of this sibling group.

However, the observer's work during the sextuplets' first three years remained unfinished until the two authors managed to give form to the extensive, detailed documentation, with all the various rhythms of life and the relational modes of this rare sibling group consisting of six same-aged children interacting with each other, their mother and other relatives present in the observations.

In chapter three the archives of that period provide the information for the psychodynamic profiles of the sextuplets. These profiles represent a model for the study of the children's psycho-affective development and a valid contribution to research projects based on *Infant Observation*, both the studies already published as well as the work in other countries described by Dina Vallino in her book *Essere Neonati (To Be a Baby)* (2004).

We find particularly interesting the separate longitudinal narratives regarding each individual sextuplet. These narratives help to distinguish each child's personality traits and facilitate the task of remembering each sextuplet individually. We read how they were perceived by the observer as based on her first impressions (see Fig. 1) that were both suggestive and pertinent to the evolutional paths described in the profiles of each child.

It is, however, in chapter four, entitled "Being in Six", that the experiences of both the observer and the discussion group find a new possibility to study in depth the history of this unusual sibling group through the individuation and interpretation of the mother/baby/sextuplet-group relationships. It is in this chapter that the two authors explain many important related aspects of the biological community that is the object of their study. They integrated descriptive, observational, listening, psychodynamic, and theoretical points of view with the different stages of development of the sextuplet group. This resulted in an interpretative vertex of the organizational processes of relational life in the first three years.

In our opinion this chapter re-confirms the validity of Esther Bick's well-defined *Infant Observation* method in this unusual situation. It also demonstrates the usefulness of the model in its containing function for all the specific aspects of this sextuplet group. Such an observational study stimulates thoughts and hypotheses regarding the group life of siblings—a topic that to date has not been sufficiently studied.

We gave wholehearted support to the observer's proposal to carry out a follow-up of this family group after the 15-year lapse, a project comprising follow-up home visits as well as administration of intellectual evaluation tests, socio-relational questionnaires, drawings, and written self-presentations prepared by the siblings. We were all motivated by a certain degree of curiosity, an important incentive in any research situation, and our minds were attentive and open to new, unexpected findings.

Thus we too found ourselves in that home, in the living room with the mother, the other relatives and the sextuplets. All of them are now young adults, each with his own personal history and particular interests, aspirations, tendencies. Each sextuplet now clearly has an individual identity, yet the six young adults are still all together as a very united group. Over the years this sibling community has transformed itself from a purely biological community into a functional community with continual relational exchanges within the group and with the outside world.

Recently, increased attention has been given to the importance of sibling experiences in the development of individual identity, including a review of the literature on this topic (D. Vallino; L. Mori). The contributions of the present study on sextuplets have led us to reflect further on certain theories regarding the sibling paradigm and the so-called sibling complex. We have noted the many other facts besides birth order which have a determining influence on the lives of the individuals in a sibling group.

We agree with our two colleagues that there are more elements of continuity than discontinuity in the comparisons between the infant profiles and the later ones. We have seen that already at the beginning of the observations there were premonitory signs of certain disturbances of development of important relational significance. These signs were evidenced in the follow-up after 15 years and predictive of areas of psychological discomfort and evolutional crises.

A follow-up aims at verifying previous findings, insofar as one looks for further information, re-examining in depth and continuing to explore the research material. In this study it was a question of acquiring further knowledge, quality- and quantity-wise, about the sextuplets. The information presented in this book is abundant and noteworthy, but we believe that it is precisely the information supplied by the follow-up that makes it so remarkable. The new input allows us to look back and reconsider the original observation experience, the work done before, including all our group discussions re-elaborating the observations. The result is an ample vision, a reflection *après-coup* on the complex infant/early childhood phase in the life of the sextuplets.

We wish to conclude these personal comments pointing out that the life of a group of six same-age siblings, which began over 20 years ago in that maternal womb with so many emotions and great courage (which truly needs to be said!), is still present today inside a sort of nest-like womb in that home to which the observer returned.

Gina Ferrara Mori and Franco Mori
Florence, Italy

# INTRODUCTION

This book presents a study on the development of a group of sextuplets. The exceptional feature of this birth received widespread attention in the media because not only were they sextuplets, but also they were born almost at term, all weighing more than a kilogram and without any serious health problems, such that they were all released from the hospital after they were two months old. The medical staff that assisted at the birth were composed of various doctors and professionals (a gynaecologist, a neonatalogist, a paediatrician, an anaesthetist, a midwife, and a nurse) to assure the care and survival of the mother and the babies, to guarantee insofar as possible their good health and a favourable beginning for their lives.

At the time of their birth in the 1980's such multiple births were rarer than they are today. The days of the rich flowering of discoveries, working methods and technological sophistication in the fields of science and medicine regarding maternity and medically assisted procreation were yet to come. Even in the field of infant research in-depth studies on child psychology, in particular regarding the innate abilities and interactive capacities of children, were still in their early stages of development.

Parallel with the progress in those fields, there was an international diffusion of Esther Bick's *Infant Observation* methodology for use in the formation of psychotherapists and child psychoanalysts. Over the years this method was extended, with the necessary adaptations, to other specific areas such as psychological diagnosis, prevention of developmental disturbances in children, and psychotherapeutic containment of parents and their young infants.

We chose to use the *Infant Observation* material in our study of these sextuplets, a rarely explored situation then and now. The results were extremely fruitful in regard to the quantity of data gathered about both the children and the organization of the family's daily life. It gave us the opportunity to investigate in depth the relational, affective and emotional aspects of the children, providing first-hand knowledge of this particular sextuplet group, allowing us to formulate hypotheses on the psycho-affective development of each child. At the end of the three-year observation period the observer, Linda Root Fortini, was aware of having had a very unusual, stimulating, and strong emotional experience, but she did not feel ready to draw up a conclusive report, as required in Esther Bick's methodology. She felt assured, however, that notwithstanding the foreseeable difficulties in managing their life in general, the family was sufficiently prepared to face the future.

There was a hibernation period of 15 years before the observer was ready to re-contact the mother. The objective was to evaluate the infant observations done through a follow-up study. Thus, the infant observations, carried out when the sextuplets were six months to three and a half years old, were completed with a research project aimed at evaluating them as they approached adulthood, by observing their individual development and the relationships among the six as well as with their parents and grandparents.

Renewing the contact with the family awakened in the observer memories of her past experience. There was a resurgence of various hypotheses and questions that had been raised during the group discussions but had not been reconsidered since then. Moved by curiosity, the observer re-read the observational reports and with surprise discovered that each child of 15 years before was recognizable in the corresponding young adult, as if that past experience had remained deposited in her unconscious and conserved in memory for the entire lapse of time. The material gathered with the *Infant*

*Observation* furnished a remarkable and important contribution to knowledge of the sextuplets and was revealed to be a useful tool for psychoanalytical research *a posteriori*.

This book consists of five chapters. The first describes the methodology. The next three chapters contain the history and synthesis of the child observations: first there is a description of the birth and the early childhood development of the sextuplets in the family environment (chapter two), then a presentation of psychodynamic profiles of each child, based on individual mother-child relationships, the mother's perception of each child, and each child's behaviour towards its parents, grandparents and the other five siblings (chapter three). The fourth chapter focuses on the development of an atypical maternal identity, the mother/baby/sextuplet group relationships, the process of psychological diversification, and the building of the individual personality within the sibling group. The fifth chapter consists of the follow-up of each child in late adolescence with an evaluation of the factors that contribute to continuity and/or discontinuity in their individual development, concluding with some thoughts about the importance of sibling relationships in personality development.

# CHAPTER ONE

# Research methods and structure

The aim of this research project is to study sibling relationships in a group of sextuplets, to observe each individual child's development and relationship with the mother as well as the mother's relationship to the sibling group as a whole.

The study was carried out in two phases using different methods. In the first phase we studied the development of the sextuplets by *Infant Observation* for the period from age six and a half months to three and a half years. The second phase focused on their development in late adolescence, from age 18 to 21 years, using various instruments, in particular projective and intelligence tests and a socio-relational questionnaire. No observations or systematic psychodynamic evaluations were done during the 15 years in-between the two phases.

The aim of the first phase of the project was to observe the sextuplet group in infancy and early childhood, in particular the relationships among these siblings and each individual child's relationship with the mother as well as with the other family members. There was a group discussion of the report presented by the observer after each of the 31 observations (including one at the nursery school and the last two at six month intervals). The method established by Esther Bick (1964) consists of observing the development of an infant in his family environment for one hour a week from birth to the age of two. The observer does not take notes during the session, but writes afterwards a detailed report of everything that has happened in chronological order. This report is then read aloud and discussed in depth in the weekly seminar, with not more than ten participants and supervised by a psychoanalyst or psychotherapist specialized in *Infant Observation*. The method involves three basic stages: 1) the observation of the child in the family situation, 2) detailed transcripts of each observation, and 3) seminar discussions in a small group. These three stages allow the observer to learn about the baby's primitive psychic world, to understand non-verbal communication, and to follow the development of the mother-child relationship.

Observing how a child develops in his family environment involves learning to stay within a particular emotional atmosphere, to observe complicated relational processes without relying on precise classifications and fixed categorizations. There is inevitably an emotional impact that the observer must learn to recognize; these strong feelings can be used in understanding his/her transference and counter-transference from which important information can be obtained. Gradually the observer learns to have an open, flexible mind, to be attentive, receptive and intuitive without participating directly so as not to influence the course of the events that take place in the family situation.

The study of these mother-baby-sextuplet group relationships required a special visiting schedule, appropriate for both the task at hand and for the family routine. Thus, Gina Ferrara Mori (the supervisor of our group) worked out adaptations to the classic *Infant Observation* method. The observational sessions lasted for two hours each (instead of the one-hour session established by Esther Bick) and took place monthly (instead of weekly) for a period of two years followed by the last two sessions at six-month intervals. These adjustments were due to the number of children involved and because the family lived in a far away town.

The reader can well imagine that the observations of the interactions of each child with the mother were continually interrupted by the numerous needs and requests of one or another of the other sextuplets. This made it difficult for the observer to pay constant attention to an individual child for adequate lengths of time. It was, however, possible to reconstruct each mother-child interaction longitudinally through the various observations and the relative group discussions.

The discussion group formed specifically for this study was composed of a neonatalogist (Corrado Vecchi), a paediatrician (Giampaolo Donzelli) who was the family paediatrician throughout the years, an auxologist (Ivan Nicoletti), a psychologist-psychotherapist with experience in *Infant Observation* (the observer, Linda Root Fortini), and two psychoanalysts, one (Gina Ferrara Mori) a paediatrician who specialized in child psychoanalysis and teacher of *Infant Observation* groups, and the other (Franco Mori) an expert in working with groups. The group met once a month to discuss the monthly observation session. Thus, six minds were involved in thinking about and delving into the observations, and this undoubtedly constituted an important support for the observer who was involved in such a complex and "overcrowded" situation.

The interdisciplinary group worked closely, well aware that this was a unique experience in the field of studies on child development. The different members, with their professional expertise, shared the interest of observing the development of the sextuplets in the family environment. It was decided to follow the sextuplets in the broadest sense possible, regarding both normal evolutional phases during the first three years of life and the relationships within the family.

When the children reached the age of one year, the seminar group felt the need to administer the Brunet-Lezine test, specifically aimed at evaluating psycho-motor development in children. Again Gina Ferrara Mori made some special adaptations so that the test could be administered in the family home on a day midway between two observation sessions. The examiner (Edda Gazzarini) carried out the test in the presence of another psychologist (Daisy Mazzetti) trained in the use of Esther Bick's method, who observed the mother-child relationship during the administration of the individual tests and subsequently wrote a detailed report of the event.

At the conclusion of the observational period, the discussion group stopped their monthly meetings and the observational reports and discussion notes were filed without further elaboration.

The paediatrician continued to monitor the physical growth of the sextuplets, with the occasional collaboration of the auxologist.

When the sextuplets turned 18 the paediatrician arranged for another physician (Filippo Filippini), who is also a psychologist, to administer projective tests. He then asked the observer to re-contact the mother and investigate the psycho-cognitive development of the sextuplets.

The test chosen was the WAIS, a well-known standard test for evaluation of individual intellectual function. The test was administered at home and assessed by two psychologists (Angela Sforza and Mario Ruocco), each of whom examined three of the sextuplets, all individually. On that occasion Linda Root Fortini, resuming partially her preceding role of observer, made the first of the three annual follow-up visits to the home; a report was written up immediately after each of these three visits. She decided to carry out a follow-up study, in collaboration with a psychologist-psychotherapist colleague, Laura Mori, to compare the development of each of the sextuplets in infancy/early childhood with that in late adolescence.

At the second follow-up visit, all the sextuplets filled out a socio-relational questionnaire prepared by the authors, and at the last visit the mother was asked to give her consent to permit the observer to carry out a retrospective study and written consents from all the members of the family were obtained. During this visit the mother gave the observer a copy of the book she had written together with a journalist about a year after the last observational visit. During the three years of the follow-up study the mother and the observer had occasional telephone conversations in which the mother talked about her children's lives, expressing her own opinions and preoccupations about them.

The authors contacted the gynaecologist, paediatricians and various psychologists who had been involved with the family to obtain information. These data, together with more obtained from other sources (including newspaper and magazine articles as well as scientific articles and information from medical meetings), were used to draw up the psychodynamic profiles of the individual sextuplets. These profiles were then discussed and investigated in depth with the two psychoanalysts who had participated in the *Infant Observation* discussions.

It was not possible to do a comparative study with similar situations in that observations on sibling groups from multiple births are rare. Only a few studies have been done on this topic but they use different methods. There have been some studies on the mother-twins relationship using the *Infant Observation* method. Still other studies have followed the pregnancy experiences of mothers of twins and/or experiences involving the intra-uterine life of the foetuses through ultrasound scans.

As far as we know there are no other catamnestic studies with such a long-term follow-up as ours.

At the last two international meetings on *Infant Observation* (Cracow, Poland in 2002 and Florence, Italy in 2004) we had the chance to compare our experience with the findings of a study on quadruplets conducted in Mexico by N. Reyes de Polanco, where, however, the observations were focused on only one of the quadruplets, rather than on the entire group, as in our case.

Our study and understanding of the individual children's development and the relationships within the sextuplet group benefited from the particular focus on individual psychodynamic profiles in two precise evolutional periods, infancy to early childhood and late adolescence, using and integrating very composite material from various sources and using different methods.

# CHAPTER TWO

# Infancy and childhood as seen through *infant observation*

*The first three numbered sections of this chapter are based on spontaneous comments made by the mother during the observations and the follow-up study as well as what she wrote in her book.*

## 1   Prehistory

The future parents met, both practically still adolescents, at a dance in a community centre. She fell in love immediately with the young man who was a good soccer player in his home-town team. They began seeing each other regularly, but only at weekends because he worked in a factory in northern Italy, and like so many young couples they had to wait to marry because of financial difficulties. Both came from farming families.

The future mother of the sextuplets is an elementary school teacher. She is a middle child in a family with three children, and describes herself as "the shadow between two brothers". She remembers having a trouble-free childhood and making dresses for her many dolls. "I took them everywhere; when I went out I often took two or three with me … maybe even six. Already then, I guess, I had what it takes to be a super-mom." After finishing the specialized high school for teachers she decided to get a university degree to be "fully qualified"; she was not satisfied with only an occupational school diploma. She was ambitious and determined and worked during the day and studied at night.

This mother is a dynamic, sociable woman. The father, an only child, is reserved, a man of few words.

Before their marriage the future mother's father became seriously ill and was diagnosed with a chronic kidney disease. Being very attached to him she felt "frightened and upset", and began to lose weight. She ended up weighing only 40 kilograms (c. 88 pounds) and stopped menstruating. As an adolescent she had often dieted, losing 23 kilos in less than two years, which was for her "a marvellous victory".

The sextuplet's maternal grandparents are dedicated to their family and "willing to sacrifice whatever is necessary to help their three children". The young couple and the sextuplets have lived with them over the years. There is little information about the paternal grandparents.

## 2    The pregnancy and birth

Before her marriage the future mother underwent, though not willingly, a series of medical examinations proposed by her gynaecologist in preparation for hormone treatment (gonadotropins) to induce pregnancy to cure her amenorrhoea. This was the beginning of the long road that led to the pregnancy and the birth of the sextuplets.

From the very beginning of the pregnancy this young woman had to change her life style: she had to follow precise medical regimens and give up her independence, as happens to many future mothers. The 17th-week ultrasound showed four or six heads, a single placenta and six choria. This news left her totally disoriented: she was practically paralysed and wordless, and felt that she lacked points of reference, terrorized as she was by the idea of a very difficult pregnancy. She recounts that at the time she was advised to get psychiatric help.

The prospect of a multiple birth with so many babies, a most exceptional event, was unthinkable: such things belong to the animal world rather than the human one. How can one face becoming the mother of a "tribe" of children all at once?

After the initial shock the mother reacted energetically, determined to go on. She later told the observer that she wanted "all or none" of them: a black and white attitude that left no room for doubts or fears, repressing an unconscious desire to have only one baby to take care of. The strong conflicts involved in this experience surfaced in a recurrent dream that she reports in her book: "I was pregnant and giving birth, and the babies died one after the other; only one lived, but it was beautiful." However, she remained optimistic, feeding on the fantasy that she was a sort of television soap opera heroine who was different from all other mothers. At the same time she was busy collecting all the information she could on multiple births.

The pregnancy was difficult because of abdominal pain, surgery for ovarian cysts, and then cervical closure by cerclage at the end of the fourth month, at which time she felt she could already be at the seventh month due to the size of her belly. Subsequently she was hospitalized and she remembered having seen many women come and go while she remained for weeks in the maternity ward. Her uterus had become enormous and her weight had increased rapidly to 80 kg (she gained a kilo a day during the last days of the pregnancy). She was unable to sleep at night, suffered from *pruritus gravidarum*, and needed six pillows to sit properly.

In her book she relates having a terrifying fantasy: "During the last period I had become another woman, and I didn't like myself anymore. My belly was abnormal, a tragicomic thing, and I was growing in all directions, in length and in width, and the rate of growth was phenomenal. I was curious to know what incredible imbalance could have taken place inside me. Where were my liver and my lungs? They certainly couldn't be where they were supposed to be. Maybe they had been pushed higher up, perhaps towards my throat. And the intestines and the kidneys? Who knows, squashed by the excess weight and ... the number of the new guests."

This multiple-foetus pregnancy set off death wishes and persecutory feelings. The mother later remembers that at a certain point she had even thought that she was "willing to die as long as the nightmare would finish", so that she could find physical and psychological relief. She was afraid that the delivery would lead to catastrophic change, potentially destructive for her own wellbeing.

Although the hospital was on alert, with a prepared staff of three gynaecologists, five anaesthetists and four paediatricians, the doctors encouraged her to be patient and to wait for a spontaneous birth because each additional day in the womb reduced the risks of premature babies. The mother, instead, hoped for a caesarean section so that she could sleep through it all, very willing to give up her role as protagonist. The normal, physiological anxieties related to giving birth, experienced to some extent by all pregnant women, become extraordinarily amplified during the waiting to give birth to six babies all at once. How could she survive?

Finally, in the middle of the winter, the event took place in a specially prepared delivery room with six incubators and a staff of six doctors. The sextuplets were born at 34½ weeks by caesarean section, and their birth weights ranged from 1200 to 1750 grams. Thus, the risks of premature delivery with very low birth weight newborns had been avoided. The newborns were all in good health, but they were put in incubators and attentively monitored and supervised in the neonatal ward for about two months.

In addition to being in good health at the time of birth, the babies probably benefited from another favourable experience: the precocious interaction among them in the womb. One could hypothesize that albeit slightly premature, they were "more mature" than other similarly premature infants because in the prenatal period they had bodily contact with their siblings and thus greater sensorial stimulations (Negri, 1994). For them birth was, thus, an experience of separation from each other as well as the mother.

## 3    Going home

The six babies remained in the hospital nursery when the mother was sent home about ten days after childbirth.

This first period was, for the mother, a temporary "ceasefire", a suspended time of waiting again for other unknowns as well as an opportunity for physical and psychological convalescence. Now that the threat of mortal danger had been overcome, there prevailed a sense of continuity of life and the mother gradually reacquired her own identity. Meantime she made long trips back and forth, almost two hours each way, to see and help take care of her babies in the hospital.

Two of the babies were scheduled to go home two months after birth, but on the designated day it was snowing and the mother was not well: "I had a fever, maybe because of my emotions." The event was postponed for a week. In one of the follow-up visits, thinking back to that period, she hypothesized that perhaps she had made the fever come on to delay the arrival of the babies.

The first two of the sextuplets to go home, Alice and Bruno, received mixed feeding, breast and bottle. Three days later the parents went to get another two babies, Daniele and Franco. Franco cried so much the first two days at home that he was taken back to the hospital and Elisa was brought home in his place. The mother maintained that she had not given Franco enough milk and that he cried out of hunger. She remembered, in the same follow-up visit mentioned above, that she had made a mistake measuring the milk powder and that the formula was not sufficient to nourish the baby. Daniele refused to take the breast by sticking out his tongue but at this point there was no more breast milk for him. Carlo was the last of the six to go home.

## 4    The first observation: "Now we are ten"

The first observation, which was also the first encounter between the observer and the mother, took place in the summer when the babies were six and a half months old.

*The grandmother, waiting at the window, announces my arrival and, immediately after, the mother opens the door with a big smile of welcome. The men of the household, the grandfather and the father, are out.* This opening scene was repeated many times over the three years of observations.

*After getting information about the frequency and duration of the observation sessions the mother and the grandmother seem satisfied and do not ask other questions. The mother talks willingly and tells how difficult things were at the beginning, but that now the children are well organized without fixed hours so "they sleep when they want".* In fact, the observer finds three of the sextuplets awake whereas the other three are still asleep in the bedroom.

*The apartment is cool and shaded and everything is clean, polished and in order. The mother and the grandmother are very cordial and conversation is easy. The mother even finds time to make a cake.* This pleasant, serene picture seems to contrast with the observer's reaction to the overcrowded entrance hall full of prams: four single ones and one double, all with pink or blue ribbons and religious medals. Then, when she sees the bedroom with the six wooden cots, each with the name of one of the babies on it, tightly jammed together to leave room for the changing table, she feels as if she is entering the nursery of a maternity ward.

*The mother says that the temperature in the bedroom must always be 24°C and that visitors are not allowed inside. Whoever wants to see the sextuplets in their room must go out onto the terrace and look at them through the window; the bedroom looks like a giant incubator. The terrace is also used as a sort of laundry area and there are nappies and bibs hanging everywhere.*

*The babies are quiet. The first sextuplet I meet is Franco who is sitting in an infant seat on the kitchen table and looking all around with interest. The mother says his name and he replies with smiles and kicks his legs. The grandmother then takes me to see Elisa, "the smallest", who is alone in the living room, lying in a carriage and playing with a rubber animal. The mother says that they were the last two babies to be born.*

*From the bedroom a baby cries and the mother goes to fetch Daniele who is awake. She brings him into the kitchen and puts him in another infant seat next to his brother. The two look at each other and coo and gurgle together. The mother doesn't say anything about Daniele.*

*After this she takes me into the bedroom to see the other three babies, who are sleeping. Alice begins to wake up at the sound of the mother's voice, and the mother says that she was the firstborn and that she is the only thumb sucker.*

*Bruno and Carlo continue to sleep.*

*The mother and the observer return to the kitchen where Franco is fussing and the grandmother picks him up and holds him in her arms.*

*Another voice is heard coming from the bedroom and the mother says it is Alice; she runs to get her and puts her in another infant seat on the floor because, different from Franco, she fears that this baby might fall from the table. She mentions the foetal position in which Alice held her arms with the elbows flexed outwards, and thinks this is probably due to trying to find enough space for herself in the womb. She adds a comment about the baby's character: "She's the only one who doesn't smile much; she's rather serious." The mother seems to have a lot to say about Alice.*

*We return to the bedroom where Carlo, the largest, is waking up. The mother says he is "withdrawn" and points out the peculiar shape of his long, narrow head, which according to her is due to the fact that "being so tight in the womb their heads were pushed one against the other". She takes him in her arms and the baby leans his head on her shoulder, closing his fists and drawing them up to himself. The mother then calls Bruno who turns towards her with big smiles and coos. She puts Carlo into the arms of the observer and picks up Bruno who gurgles looking at her. She says that he is the only one of the sextuplets who is able to stay sitting up.*

*The mother and the observer take these two babies into the kitchen.*

*It is getting close to mealtime. For now they are spoon-fed only at lunch; in the evening they get a bottle because it is quicker. The mother ties back her long hair and takes Franco to change him.*

*The doorbell rings and the "other mothers" arrive. The sister-in-law takes Franco and the mother carries Daniele into the bedroom to change him. Then she changes the two girls, meanwhile talking about her husband who has found a job near home and can now help with the children. In the morning he bottle feeds one and at lunch helps with another; in the evening he helps again. She says that, according to the father, Franco is jealous when she takes care of the other babies.*

*The mother is aware that the grandmother is good at spoon-feeding, whereas she loses her patience. Now the apartment is full of movement and chatter, and babies eating, making noise and playing.*

## 5   Organization of an enlarged family

When the babies were all home from the hospital the four-member family became a family of ten with more children than adults.

So many babies with so many needs demands a well-organized household. The mother reacts by increasing her hyperactivity in an attempt to keep everything under control and not feel overcome. This means that daily life must continue to flow as smoothly as before in a clean, orderly house with space, albeit reduced, for each member of the family. The mother relies on her experience as an elementary school teacher who knows how to handle a group of children and, at the same time, how to follow the progress of each one and respond to each individual's practical needs. She is able to recognize their differences and their potential gifts, and tries to treat them all fairly and in the same manner. Even the smallest sign of rebellion on the part of the children against her maternal authority would be disastrous for her as well as for the entire family group.

Consequently the family model must be based on efficiency, and this inevitably limits the possibilities for establishing close relationships. Meltzer (1984) used the term "maternal service" to describe the relational modality that mothers use for rapid problem solving related to children's physical needs (such as nose blowing), instead of creating emotional contacts that imply intimacy and dependence. At one point the grandmother says outright that they need someone assigned specifically to help the children blow their noses! (10th observation, 15 months).

While the mother comes and goes like a busy "Minister of Foreign Affairs", the grandmother is always present; it is she who prepares all the meals and is always available physically and emotionally as if she were the "Assistant for Affection".

By delegating the grandmother to exercise certain functions of care taking that imply dependence on bonds and emotional involvement, the mother seems to distance herself from the painful part of the maternal function. While the grandmother is the depositary of intimate one-to-one relationships, the mother dedicates herself to being the good teacher who takes note and makes the most of the developmental capacities of each individual sextuplet. How else could a mother deprived of the possibility of a deep relationship with a single child find gratification?

From the role of a super-assisted first-time mother she is transformed into a super-mother, practically a "movie star". The extraordinary event of the birth of healthy sextuplets attracts the curiosity and interest of the outside world and the mother becomes a public figure: she appears on television, gives interviews and does advertising for baby products. Hence another method of survival is to belong to the "public domain" and to look outward.

The father is a meek, quiet person. He is affectionate and patient with the children, but seems a bit disoriented and insecure. The grandfather maintains his position as head of the family. Both the father and the grandfather are home at weekends; they do not really substitute for the various women who come in regularly to help take care of the babies, but rather exercise the adjunctive role of affectionate adults who give their support to the family as a whole.

The general impression is that of a family governed by a competent pair, the grandmother and the mother who are capable of managing difficult situations and offer protection. The family has a matriarchal structure with two distinct classes, a dominant female one and a peripheral male one. These two females, assisted by neighbours and two women sent by the welfare office, are the ones who get things done and hold the power.

In their study on the educational role of the family, Meltzer and Harris (1983) describe the matriarchal family as being based on the strength and vitality of the woman alongside a less present and less adequate father figure. Such a family structure can become a "female band" if the female strength is characterized by hostility towards males or it can function as a "family-couple" if the woman has bisexual character and behavioural attributes, such as ability and strength, and thus incorporates the paternal functions.

From the very beginning the mother exercised the role of "super-parent", assisted by the grandmother, an efficient pair who know how to manage a group of children and organize the family. At times they unite to disqualify the father and mock his parental capabilities. Subsequently, when the mother is overcome by an accumulation of physical tiredness and psychological stress, she turns to her husband in a different way, requesting his help and involving him directly in the care of the children. The father figure thus acquires value and the parental couple is established.

We wish to point out, also, that the maternal grandparents, a complementary, non-antagonistic parental couple, give fundamental support to the parents of the sextuplets. The interior resources of the young parental couple appear more fragile than those of the grandparents as a couple; the latter appear better able to function emotionally at an introjective level.

## 6   The first differences

As long as the six babies could all be considered as having pretty much the same needs and could be treated as a homogeneous nestling-group, without individual behavioural problems or special needs, the adult caretakers were able to manage them fairly easily as a group, through rapid, targeted actions involving them all in a global, panoramic sense.

As time passes different individual paces of development become evident, leading inevitably to changes that threaten to destabilize and create obstacles in the daily routine. The description of how the night-time problem is solved, using camping cots, gives the impression that a new emergency is underway. The mother explains the night-time organization with easy-to-move cots, "used to bring the children into [her] bedroom during the night so that they can be rocked back to sleep when they wake up and cry, which happens often" (10 months).

As their first birthday approaches the children begin to occupy more space and require more attention. It is now practically impossible to manage them all together in the same way. They catch the flu and have fevers, sleeping problems, intestinal upsets and food intolerances. Then they begin to walk and to fuss with each other. At about the same time they begin teething.

When any one of the children seems to require special attention, has a particular need or wants a privileged relationship, the mother worries that anarchy may break out. To keep the situation in hand, she establishes a general rule for all adults (family, friends, visitors, helpers), "Don't bother the children when they are tranquil."

The children, instead, seem to adhere spontaneously to a community style regime. For example, when they are about ten months old, they all have a bowel movement at the same time of day, usually in the morning.

From the fourth observation on it is the grandmother who receives the observer because the mother begins arriving later; she is always busier and in a rush. The first signs of persecutory feelings in the mother begin to appear. She is afraid that the helpers furnished by the welfare office, two women who take turns with the children for a total of eight hours a day, are going to be curtailed. She tells the observer that they need more "hands" than "eyes", making the observer feel (in her counter-transference) alone, useless, and somewhat of a bother. The mother points out that "here everyone does something" and wants to know what is being observed (eighth observation, 13½ months).

In this very unusual situation the adults cannot be allowed to prefer or show favouritism to any of the sextuplets, and only limited time is available for any individual problem. The children spend almost all their time with each other, and the fact that they are six begins to become the "background noise" (Coles, 2003) that accompanies them throughout their growing up and is a part of each individual's experience of the self.

## 7    The first birthday

In this period the mother relives various events and experiences reactions that emphasize the problematic aspects of motherhood. To maintain her own self-esteem this super-mother finds information about other cases of multiple pregnancies; she compares the different experiences and exchanges information with mothers in other countries, even as far away as Japan and South Africa. There is evidence of strong feelings of ambivalence. For example, in the fifth observation (10½ months), during which she is mostly absent because first she is out doing the shopping and then when she comes home she decides to go to the bank, she scolds the grandmother for having put a chair in front of the wood stove to keep the children away from it, and exclaims: "It would be better for a child to be burned up … we have six of them."

The mother's thoughts sometimes become oppressive and desperate: she complains that "one can't even get sick" (meaning, have one's own needs). Although, as we have seen, she buries her depressive experiences under an omnipotent ideal self, as a public figure and famous star, she is forced to take a medical leave of absence from her teaching.

In the seventh observation the observer learns that the children's first birthday had been more an occasion for public recognition of the sextuplets, celebrated with a publicity event (the source of indispensable income), than an intimate family celebration. The mother talks about it with the observer only in reference to the need to renew the request for welfare assistance. The grandmother shows very different emotions when she mentions briefly and solemnly that "at this time a year ago we were very worried".

In the following months the mother, on leave, stays at home with the children whom she has chosen not to send to a day care nursery. The children and the adults get the flu one after another. The observer is greeted with protests and crying, in particular by Alice and Franco, whereas the other four "have just finished crying and maybe need changing", but the mother decides not to intervene. The grandmother adds: "This is quite a difficult time …" (12½ months).

The construction of the new bigger house, on two floors with five bedrooms and three bathrooms, is delayed because of the bad winter weather. Also, the family needs a means of transport large enough to accommodate all of them together.

The mother seems to be continually more apathetic and disconsolate and the house more in disorder. She remembers that "when I didn't have children the tantrums of my friends' children bothered me terribly". She says she needs to sleep more and remembers that as a girl she did not sleep much. "I would wake up and look around for sweets. I didn't eat much during the day, I was skinny. My grandmother kept the sweets locked up."

The mother's words and behaviour in this period seem to indicate a condition of delayed post-partum depression.

In another observation as the mother greets the observer she announces: "We're going out," because, she explains, "if we don't keep them outside they cause trouble!" (ninth observation, 14 months). Recently it has been impossible to take them out because going out requires at least three adults. She does not say it explicitly, but she makes it clear that she needs the observer's help. This is one of the rare times that the mother expresses a real need and communicates a sense of defeat and exhaustion without denying it. In regard to countertransference, the observer feels almost grateful to be finally "useful".

## 8    The father

The father has not been present much from the beginning of the observations. He appears only for brief moments, silent and with a style of his own. While the mother "directs the domestic traffic" he behaves like the "bus driver", proceeding slowly, cautiously, respectfully, all the while maintaining affectionate contact with all the children.

We all know the importance that the presence of parents with two distinct roles has for children's psychic health. This father does not appear to be an assistant or mere stand-in for the mother, nor a substitute or a photocopy. He exercises a different role; he is a second object, stable, and differentiated (Gaddini, 1974) who evidences so-called "weak" aspects inclined to tenderness and care taking capabilities. He manages to create a relational space of delicate intimacy with each child.

In the first observation the mother mentioned that her husband thinks that Franco is jealous when she pays attention to the other children: a comment that indicates the father's clear perception of this child's gender, as well as being in projective identification with him.

From the third observation on one begins to see a particular relationship between the father and Alice; they seek each other's company. This relationship will be significant in the girl's development (see chapter III, psychodynamic profiles).

Subsequently, during that winter of depression in which the mother is no longer able to direct the traffic, the father has more time at home with the children, and they often go to him. He is more present even during the observations. Sometimes the mother, out of desperation and with the grandmother's complicity, teases her husband. For example, when he gets sick she criticizes him saying, "With the excuse that he has flu, he stays in bed!" (eighth observation). Although she seems to give little consideration to what he does and to deride him, she could not manage without him and she permits him to exercise his father function.

As Winnicott said many years ago during a BBC radio interview, it may be difficult for the mother to choose when to call in the father, and she must permit him to exercise his function, although the realization and richness of the relationship established does not depend only on her; it depends greatly on the father and the children themselves (Winnicott, 1945). One can, thus, hypothesize that the father figure was experimented with and created by each individual sextuplet and that he was considered not only as an extension or substitute of the mother (Fairbairn, 1944).

During a walk with the children at the ninth observation (14 months) we see how the father begins to subtly extend his sphere of influence.

*As soon as the observer arrives, the mother, tired and apathetic, announces to everyone, "Today we're going out." The children are placed in pairs in the three double push-chairs. Bruno and Alice are assigned to the father, and Daniele and Franco to the observer, while Elisa and Carlo are with the mother, who says, "We never go out all together. Usually someone takes one of the children when there is an errand to run or when I go out I take two at a time."*

*The large group walks in silence. The mother has a faraway look, lost in emptiness, and the father, walks slowly and tends to remain behind. We go to see the work just begun on the foundations of the new house. When the father catches up with the group it is time to turn back. The mother, noticing that Alice is leaning forward, goes to sit her straight and then takes that push-chair from the husband who takes over the one with Elisa and Carlo. Suddenly Bruno protests and the father asks, using his nickname* (see chapter III, paragraph 2, motor difficulties), *"What's wrong, broken head?" The mother lets go of the push-chair, leaving it for her husband, adding, "Each to his own," to explain what she considers Bruno's odd behaviour. Again the father remains behind pushing Bruno and Alice.*

In the 19th observation (24 months) the mother-father-children relational situation is evident. The mother favours the contacts between the children and the father, but when the latter takes autonomous initiatives she criticizes him and the grandmother seems to echo her.

*Bruno is playing with a wooden box with holes for different geometric-shaped pieces. Suddenly Franco gets off the little car he is playing on, goes to his brother and forcefully takes the toy away. Bruno protests and yells, "Box"(pronouncing the word well). Franco continues to pull, but Bruno doesn't let go. The mother tries to get Franco interested in another box that she offers him. At the same time Bruno manages to break free from his brother's hold, at which Franco throws himself onto the floor and kicks violently, hitting the mother who complains. Carlo notices the box and he wants it, too. There is another fight and this time Bruno loses and cries. Franco has finished his tantrum and goes over to Daniele and hits him.*

*The mother announces the father's arrival, "Daddy's here." The children crowd around him with their faces turned upward searching for his attention. The father bends over slowly and gives kisses and caresses here and there in the little crowd. Then he squats down and three of the children come closer. Franco sits between his legs to be hugged and Carlo and Daniele stand next to him demanding the same.*

*Then the children follow the father into the kitchen [... .] He offers each one a piece of cookie that has been dipped in his coffee with milk ... . Seeing this, the mother expresses her disapproval and thinks it is wrong to give them something to eat so close to their mealtime. The father says nothing but continues to nibble on some cookies, sharing them with the children. The mother disappears into the bedrooms without saying anything else. Soon after the grandmother turns to Daniele, who appears to be very satisfied, and asks with a touch of sarcasm, "Now can you please*

*tell me why you won't eat your meat?", and walks out of the kitchen with
Carlo in her arms.*

*When the father has finished he goes back to the living room to smoke
a cigarette. The children follow him, each one occupied with something.
Daniele is searching for a car in the pile of toys, then looks at his father,
who understands and finds it for him. Bruno listens to music on the radio.
Carlo takes the box previously fought over, and Franco moves around in the
little car hitting against the wall at the end of each lap. Then, when he sees
Carlo playing with the box he jumps out of the car and tries to take it away
from him. Unsuccessful he picks up a potty, hits it against a cabinet and
then against the door. The father looks at him, shakes his finger and, repeats,
calmly and seriously, "No." Franco stops and, remaining immobile, as if
hypnotized, looks at his father. Then the father explains that the thing he
has in his hand is for doing pooh-pooh. Also Bruno tries to take the box from
Carlo, but again the father says a solemn "No" and Bruno desists suddenly
and lies down on the marble floor with his face turned in the opposite direction from his father's.*

The mother, who needs to go out of the house more and more
frequently, assigns the father the important role of driver of the family van.

In the 22nd observation (two years and two months), while the
father is getting the children together to put them back in the van at
the end of a jaunt, the mother tells the observer, "Things go better
when my husband is around. He has more authority and, also, since
he isn't with the kids so much he puts up with them much better
than I do: he's more patient than I am." All in all she prefers him to
the helper sent by the welfare office.

The children now benefit from the good functioning of not only
the mother-grandmother pair, but also the parental couple who take
care of other needs. With the father's full acquisition of his own position and specific role, the adults in the household become a stable,
consolidated group ready to take on the ever-greater task of raising
the children.

## 9   Objective proof of differences

When the children are about 14½ months old, the members of
the discussion group who follow their development decide it is
necessary to administer the Brunet-Lezine test to compare the

children's psycho-motor development. The test is carried out in the home halfway between two observations. The examiner is assisted by another psychologist who observes and transcribes everything that happens during the tests. Each child is tested individually, held in the mother's arms, while the father and grandmother take care of the other five in another room. The schedule is to test three in the morning and the other three in the afternoon. The mother decides the succession for the tests (Franco, Alice, Daniele, Carlo, Bruno, Elisa), but then without warning squeezes Carlo into the morning session just after the third test, because "there's still a little more time". In the afternoon Bruno refuses to submit to the test, so the mother changes the order and Elisa is presented first.

Each child evidences a very personal style, both cognitively as well as in how it relates to the mother and the examiner. Globally the test evidences a medium-high IQ, except for Carlo who cannot be evaluated because he seems afraid and cries too much to be tested. The individual results will be examined in chapter three.

## 10    Scenes from everyday life

We have selected a few particular situations that indicate the different ways in which the family members cope with and adapt to the realities of daily life.

### Lunchtime

The mother who worries about the children's development, possible sicknesses, protests, and inevitable jealousies perceives, the sextuplets at times as a threat: a persecutory group that implies a risk of mutiny and, for her, that of being shipwrecked. Every so often one gets the feeling that her negation of the difficulties of being a supermother might someday collapse.

The midday meal, that precedes the guaranteed truce of the two-hour nap, involves remarkable effort and coordination on the part of the adults who need to be alert, quick, and efficient.

Usually when the mother returns home with the children the grandmother has prepared the meal, the helper is already there, and a next-door neighbour arrives just in time. While the mother cleans and changes two children, the grandmother and the other women feed the other four, who will be cleaned up afterwards. Everything is done quickly, with concentrated determination and without time for taking a breath. The rotation of feeding and cleaning goes ahead despite hitches; for example, if one child does not want the pasta, a substitute (bread or cheese) is offered immediately, and if the child refuses that as well then the feeder skips on to the next child.

## 4th observation (nine and a half months)

*The mother decides to begin preparing the lunch and goes towards the kitchen. The helper and the neighbour arrive together. The mother picks up Daniele because he is tired and takes him to be changed. The helper and the grandmother attend to Franco and Alice. Elisa begins to cry. Bruno is on the ground playing, paying no attention to what is happening around him. Daniele is fed quickly by the grandmother and Franco by the helper. Alice is in the corner waiting to be fed by the grandmother. All three children eat seated in child seats.*

*Daniele falls asleep as soon as he has eaten. The mother gives Franco to the observer. Alice takes a long time to eat, wriggling and fussing happily and the grandmother responds with the same tone. Then she gives the little girl a drink of water.*

*The mother directs the traffic, never stopping for a moment. She puts Daniele to bed and in his place takes Bruno and gives him to the helper; she puts Franco to bed and takes Elisa. Only Carlo does not eat because he is already asleep. "He'll eat when he wakes up," the mother says.*

## 7th observation (12½ months)

*The neighbour arrives and immediately picks up Franco, her favourite. The grandmother takes Alice into her arms, kisses her and goes to change her. Then, in the kitchen the mother is already feeding Daniele and in the next room the neighbour is feeding Franco. Carlo is moving around, looking at his brother in the infant seat; he hits his hand against the chair but doesn't seem to realize it and seems not to be hungry. The helper puts Bruno in the infant seat and feeds him. Meantime the grandmother is feeding Alice. Elisa plays alone in the living room.*

*The neighbour says Franco is not eating much and the grandmother replies that he is probably sleepy and suggests giving him his fruit together with the pasta. Then the grandmother opens the drawer with the knives and forks to distract Alice so that she can feed her more quickly. Daniele eats tranquilly while he plays with his mother's necklace.*

*"They don't drink enough," observes the grandmother and she gives the little girl some water. Franco does not finish his food, then he and Alice are put to bed.*

*The helper goes to the living room to get Carlo and the grandmother takes Elisa. They are the last to eat.*

Here we see that the mealtime rhythm is quicker than before. The children have more needs and the adults less time. The grandmother's statement about the children not drinking enough suggests that things should be slowed down, that there should be pauses in the feeding, and that perhaps someone should think about individual needs.

## 20th observation (26 months)

*There is movement in the entrance hall. Carlo, in the neighbour's arms, does not want to be put down. Daniele is sitting on the kitchen table. Alice brings her still full plate into the kitchen. Bruno wanders around aimlessly.*

*The grandmother takes Elisa and puts her in the highchair. Alice begins to call her repeatedly, "Eli, Eli". The grandmother feeds Elisa brusquely, asking Alice if she wants a taste, but Alice refuses categorically and goes away. Bruno spills a glass of egg whites and the mother scolds him severely. Daniele leans forward in his seat on the table to see what has happened; then he plays, dangerously, with a glass that the mother has left near the edge of the table. Elisa smudges her face and hair with pasta, and the grandmother, irritated, offers her some water that the little girl pours on the highchair tray. The grandmother scolds her loudly and complains in despair about the situation in general.*

*The neighbour has to go home to prepare lunch for her own family and leaves Carlo crying. The mother takes Daniele, the helper Franco and the grandmother Elisa to change them. Franco does not want to be cleaned by the helper. The mother quickly finishes with Daniele and takes Franco who stops crying. Daniele, whose shoes are being untied by the helper, begins to fuss. The grandmother takes Elisa into the bedroom telling her to say goodbye to the observer. Bruno begins yelling because Carlo is pulling his hair. Subsequently, Carlo begins to cry because Bruno tries to take revenge, and there are cries of pain. The mother orders the two children to stop. The helper tries to take Daniele into the bedroom but he cries and kicks his legs. Alice walks to the bedroom by herself. The mother prepares the usual treat of sweets to give them when they are all in bed.*

As the months pass mealtimes become more and more chaotic because what are normal needs for a child must be multiplied by six. The mother's quandary is understandable, and in her book she says that she remembers the good old times "when the children were all around me at the table and with a single dish and a single spoon I gave them their meal. In about five minutes they all had had enough to eat and were ready to go to sleep. Changing them was practically a delight! It was like a production chain: we would lay them all down in a row on the table in the kitchen or in the hall or even on the floor and change them one after another. Back then they didn't care if I changed them or someone else did ... . To convince them to go to bed for their afternoon nap ... I had to offer a treat: I gave them something sweet, they called them 'Mummy's sweeties'. Then, to be sure they were all safe I would lock the door and they didn't fuss because they didn't realize they were prisoners."

### Different care taking styles

When the children are all at home together, the grandmother separates them into pairs or groups.

### 7th observation (12½ months; the mother is out)

*As soon as the observer arrives the grandmother informs her, as if to show how good she is with them, that the children have all been playing for two hours without asking for attention. She has divided them in pairs in three play-pens in the living room: Alice is with Daniele, Bruno with Carlo, Elisa with Franco. The latter two have big smiles for the observer when they see her. Then Franco plays peek-a-boo with her, turning his face away.*

*Alice is pretty much by herself, standing up and leaning on the side of the play-pen with her thumb in her mouth. The helper takes Bruno in her arms and Carlo begins to cry. "See," says the grandmother, "you shouldn't have picked him up. Now they'll all want to be picked up." The helper defends herself: "But, he was crying." The grandmother points out that the children are jealous of each other. She gives Carlo a biscuit, but he refuses it and she then takes him into her arms. The helper puts Bruno back in the*

*play-pen and the grandmother gives Carlo to her. Bruno begins to cry deso-*
*lately, sitting with his shoulder against the net of the play-pen and his face*
*half-hidden behind his arm. Franco goes back and forth inside his play-pen*
*while continuing to smile at the observer. The grandmother puts Elisa in*
*a baby-walker and goes to telephone the mother. Alice and Daniele are sit-*
*ting in their play-pen throwing toys here and there; their legs are touching*
*and they are gurgling. Alice looks cheerfully at the observer and lowers her*
*head towards her shoulder a bit coquettishly. The helper puts Bruno and*
*Carlo in two other walkers. The three children move all around bumping*
*into each other. Daniele sees them, stands up and tries to climb up the side*
*of the play-pen. He cries a little. Alice stands up, too, and starts sucking*
*the edge of the play-pen while Daniele, agitated and angry, moves close and*
*pushes her. Alice moves away but he comes close again and gives her a push*
*with his head.*

In the course of another observation one can see how the mother behaves with the children before going out and when she comes home.

## 10th observation (15 months)

*Before going out the mother quickly puts a lot of toys in the living room,*
*offering something to each child to keep it occupied while she is gone. She*
*gets ready to go out, puts her sunglasses on Alice, who makes a show of*
*it. Franco is interested in a toy, and Carlo whines sitting astraddle on the*
*floor paying no attention to the things around him. Bruno watches the*
*mother while she gets her wallet and leaves. Then Daniele comes out from*
*the kitchen and surveys the toys on the floor. Elisa is out with her favourite*
*of the helpers.*

*When the mother returns almost an hour later, she seems dazed, lost*
*in her thoughts, and has difficulty in renewing contact with the children*
*and establishing an empathic feeling. The children run all around her*
*and she, afraid of being overcome and wanting to stop them, tells them*
*to stamp their feet on the floor. But they don't do it. So then the mother*
*takes a paper bag, blows it up and hits it to make it burst, as if to stun*
*them.*

Whereas when she went out, the mother knew what to do: give each child a toy, when she returned home it was more difficult for her to re-adjust and she tries to keep the group of children at a distance.

11th observation (16 months)

*The grandmother is alone with the children and the helper because the mother had to go to her school. The grandmother complains that the school authorities show little understanding of the mother's difficult situation. She informs the observer that the previous Sunday the parents had gone out alone for a few hours. The grandmother thinks that the children are restless* (maybe she, too, feels the absence of her daughter). *She decides to do a sort of test: she asks repeatedly, out loud, "Where's Mamma?" She adds that all six can say the word "Mamma", but the word "Babbo"* (Daddy in Italian) *is more difficult. The four boys immediately stare at the front door. Bruno's eyes remain fixed on the door for a few minutes, but the two girls do not appear to be interested in the question. Elisa is in the arms of her favourite helper; Alice seems not to have any reaction, and then she takes two wooden blocks and goes over to the grandmother and hits the blocks together very hard.* (This reminds us of symbolic play, like the spool game described by Freud in which she expresses her desire to have a favourite carer all to herself.)


12th observation (17 months; the grandmother is out)

*The mother is alone with the helper and five of the children. Alice has been sent to the beach with the grandparents. The mother tells the observer that she is taking advantage of this unusual situation to make some changes in the domestic routine: she has decided to "re-educate" Elisa and Franco to put them in line with the other sextuplets' sleeping habits since they both have particular problems going to sleep, and the grandmother defends these individual needs. Elisa wants to be cradled by the grandmother before going to sleep and Franco wakes in the night and then goes to sleep in the grandparents' bed with them.*

During this observation the mother appears anxious, dissatisfied, and suspicious about the help from the helper and the neighbour.

*After a phone call from the grandmother she is less uneasy and more relaxed: she stops reproaching the helper who is holding Elisa in her arms. Right after contacting the grandmother she remembers to offer coffee to the observer, a hospitable gesture that the grandmother usually makes.*

In the above series of events we see the mother's ambivalent feelings regarding the grandmother's absence. On one hand there seems to be some rivalry with her own mother (she wants to change the bedtime "rules"), on the other she feels the grandmother's absence, and she does not trust the substitutes. For the first time, as if she too feels the absence of the grandmother, the observer intervenes to warn the mother that one of the children has a piece of plastic in his mouth (an indication of her counter-transference).

While saying good-bye at the end of the observation, the mother becomes hoarse, a common condition among teachers, and a problem she says she has had since the birth of the sextuplets. "I hate it when I lose my voice," as if this deficiency might express symbolically her fear of not being able to manage on her own.

When the grandparents and Alice return from the beach, the mother declares solemnly and without a moment of hesitation that "None of the children should get used to being an only child." There can not be preferences, privileges, or special treatment: the group must march forward united and compact! (18 months).

## 11   The second year: "The children are everywhere!"

Feeling overcome by her maternal duties and resigned to her "school" group's need for full-time care, at the end of the summer the mother decides to ask to extend her leave of absence from teaching and later to make a specific request to work as a substitute teacher rather than full-time. She is forced to face reality and take less refuge in the maniacal defence of being a super-mother.

The children are a year and a half old; they are all walking and can go up and down stairs. In fact they go wherever they want! The sides are taken off the cots so that they can learn to get in and out of bed by themselves. The apartment becomes progressively smaller and more uncomfortable. The adults have accumulated months and months of mental stress and physical fatigue. It is no longer possible to depend on a unified rhythm of psychomotor development and the difficulties of managing them all together increase exponentially. Now, when they go out, one or another of the children refuses to stay the whole time in the pram.

Each child begins gradually to demonstrate his own individual personality and temperament and behavioural characteristics.

Alice tends to be a little lady, imitating the mother and the grandmother.

Bruno, who keeps his mother's whereabouts under scrutiny, often plays all by himself.

Carlo has violent temper tantrums, banging his head against anything at the height of his rage.

Daniele is very agile, always in motion, climbing up and down, even dangerously so; he usually has a dummy in his mouth.

Elisa is easy-going, inquisitive and friendly; she is very willing to have substitute carers.

Franco is assertive and original in his play, and friendly like Elisa; he is the baby a neighbour prefers.

Up to now the "barracks" style regimen, based on restrictions and prohibitions, has worked well enough. For example, the children are not allowed to feed themselves, because "that would mean at least half an hour for each one … ", and the day would be taken up with mealtimes.

At a certain point each child tends to do his own thing and the regimen of controls and prohibitions has a disintegrating effect that risks leading to just what the mother fears most: rebellion or mutiny. Even the neighbours recognize that the mother's many problems are sixfold.

In September the situation is chaotic, difficult to cope with, and on the verge of madness. The 15th observation (20 months) begins with the mother yelling furiously and in open conflict with Elisa.

*She explains to the observer, who has barely entered the house, that the little girl "doesn't want to be changed! OK, then she'll stay wet with pee-pee!". Elisa, crying and very pale, is having a tantrum and the mother is trying to prepare to go out before the other children begin to fuss too. She asks the observer if it is raining, worried about the weather but anxious to take the children out.*

*The walk calms things down for a bit, but afterwards the mother is once again uneasy. She asks the observer to take Elisa, who is trying to get out of the push-chair; crying, Elisa wriggles and kicks and refuses to stand up. The mother says, "If you don't stop it we'll go crazy … you ugly, little, skinny thing!" and then rushes into the house to wash her hair. She returns with a towel on her head and wearing a white smock, ready to face mealtime.*

In this episode the mother seems to express, on one hand, the desire to wash away and out of her hair problems and preoccupations that are crowding her mind and, on the other, the need to find within herself sufficient professional ability (by wrapping herself in a doctor's white coat) to manage emergencies without getting emotionally overwhelmed.

In the next observation (21 months) the family atmosphere is completely different: everyone is calm, the father is there, and the mother decides that they should all go for a ride in the new van. This makes it possible for her to experience a pleasant and consolatory moment of regression. Perhaps the mother can let herself go, fantasizing about being a teacher with a chauffeur, a couple in harmony and well equipped to carry out parental tasks.

Again in the 19th observation (24 months) both parents are present with the sextuplets. They are all together in the living room and the mother brings the observer up to date on the most recent event: Franco broke the glass on the front door, but they have decided it is not worth repairing even though the new house is not yet ready.

The father appears very "patient", as the mother descotes him, because "he isn't home much". The father demonstrates his ability to maintain discipline and to say no. He is at ease with the children and willing to be involved, less disturbed by the children's tantrums and knows how to stop their misbehaviour. He is comfortable with the children as a group. The mother, instead, intervenes in a different way: she tries to distract the children, to offer a substitute in consolation, and even plays the role of a group animator, organizing recreational activities to keep them occupied and out of trouble's way.

*The mother is seated on the floor with the children all around her ... . All of a sudden she jumps up and organizes a group exercise session* (17th observation, at 22 months).

*After having told the observer the latest news about the children and shown her an article about them just published in a well-known magazine, the mother calls the children with enthusiasm and has them form a circle, announcing that it is dance time* (18th observation, at 23 months).

In the 22nd observation (27 months) she organizes a singing lesson.

Although the good weather means that the children can stay outside and take trips in the van, the family atmosphere reflects tiredness and discouragement. The grandmother is worried because the children do not want to use the potty. "They stand in the corners and do it in their nappies and then come to us to be changed." She adds that if they do not learn they will not be accepted at the nursery school in September.

Again at the 23rd observation (28 months), the grandmother complains that the children still have not learned to control their bladder and bowel movements: they play in the garden without nappies doing their pee-pee everywhere.

*The grandmother is sitting with Carlo on her lap next to the observer. Seeing Bruno play with the potty, she announces in a loud voice, "The potty is for doing pooh-pooh. You don't have to do it now, just call Grandma when you need to go." She says that her own children stopped dirtying themselves when they were about a year old, but the sextuplets don't say anything until after they have done it. She feels desperate about their indifference and adds, "They're little rascals; they don't even have an afternoon nap anymore." She tells the observer that the day before in the bedroom they broke a ceiling lamp that she had had for more than 40 years. Someone had thrown a toy up in the air and pieces of glass rained down everywhere, on the floor, on the beds, into their hair. "It could have been very dangerous. There must be someone up there who protects them … otherwise, by now … ."*

*The mother, exhausted and beside herself, asks, "What can we do?… nothing works." She realizes that things are better when her husband is there because "he has more authority and puts up with things better", whereas she is "tired".*

In mid-August (30 months) the grandmother agrees to take care of the children while the parents go away to the seaside for four days, although at the last minute the mother is unsure about going. It rains the whole time, making it seem a useless attempt at relaxing and getting away from the exhausting family routine. Then, almost a confirmation of the mother's worry about going away, the grandmother says that it was a terrible experience at home: "The children did pooh-pooh in their pants, dirtying everything, even the walls. It took two hours to clean up and the smell was still there!"

Everything's exploding, and nothing can be held together.

In September the family moves into the new house.

The grandmother says that the sextuplets all go to nursery school, staying for lunch, but they do not sleep at night. The mother has gone back to teaching; she has a fourth grade class with only five students. "There have been so many changes, poor things; let's hope they'll get used to it all quickly because some nights we don't get any sleep."

The father takes the observer around the new house, with the children in tow. The mother is very busy preparing for the arrival of her brother and his children and another family with quadruplets. The new house is already chock-full of people.

When the mother finally slows down, she tells the observer that she has been having a disagreement with her colleagues at the nursery school because they advise waiting a few more months before sending Carlo with the others. She appears alarmed and unhappy about this: "They wanted to talk to me alone to ask me not to send Carlo with them to kindergarten until January. I used to be worried about him, I thought he was deaf ... instead what he really needs is to socialize .... How can I keep him home alone? First of all, that's just what he wants. Then in January, he'll refuse to go to nursery school again. Elisa, for example, had to stay home for a few days because of an intestinal upset, but she couldn't bear staying home alone; for her it was practically a punishment." (To acknowledge a personal need of any of the children is always a threat for the mother.)

After this angry outburst, the observer feels dazed and overpowered by the new events (moving to the new house, the nursery school and another super-mother with quadruplets) and in her counter-transference feels as if everything was beginning all over again instead of leading towards a conclusion.

## 12    Observation at the nursery school

The observation takes place on a Saturday when there are normally fewer children and those present are kept in a single group with two teachers. The sextuplets are usually divided, with three in each class: Elisa, Bruno and Carlo in one and Alice, Daniele and Franco in the other.

*Elisa is the first to see the observer and smiles at her. Bruno goes close to his sister and, holding on to her shoulder, looks very seriously at the observer. Franco is near the window drawing. Daniele and Alice are sitting next to each other at a table together with other children, and they are all drawing. Carlo is sitting on the top of the same table with one hand in the other and his legs hanging down. The younger teacher is in front of him and he isn't doing anything. He stares at the observer for a long time.*

*The other teacher is picking up pieces of a construction set. She asks out loud if anyone has taken a black screw that is missing. Bruno, who is sitting next to Franco, timidly holds up a plastic wheel with the screw in it; he looks at her, but says nothing. The teacher doesn't notice and continues her search. Bruno lowers his hand and turns the screw around in the wheel until the teacher sees him and exclaims, "There it is! Bruno has it." He gives it to her and watches what she does with it. Then he looks at the observer again and after that kneels down and plays with the construction set.*

*Franco takes the younger teacher's hand to be accompanied to the bathroom.*

*Carlo, all by himself, begins to cry, looking around in distress. The other teacher calls him, and then puts him on the floor, encouraging him to find a toy.*

*Daniele gets off his chair and goes to get a bunch of figure cards. Alice, who was sitting next to him, also stands up and walks around the room with a notebook under her arm staring at the observer. Daniele, with lots of figure cards, runs towards the observer but bumps into another boy and some of the cards fall on the floor. Daniele picks up what he can, while Alice confronts the other boy and says, "No," raising her arm threateningly. Then she runs after her brother and hits the first child she meets along the way.*

*Franco has found a small toy pistol that he shows to everyone, pretending to shoot here and there. Elisa and Bruno immediately go near him and then also Alice and Daniele. They all want the pistol. The sibling group is recomposed except for Carlo who is still crying.*

*The teacher decides that the children must take turns using the pistol and Franco waits patiently until all his siblings have had a chance to play with it. As soon as he gets it back he "shoots" at the teacher, who plays along and pretends to fall. The children seem happy to play with their brother Franco.*

*Carlo continues to cry. He slowly approaches the observer, raising his arms to be picked up, and looks at her sadly. The observer says, "Carlo is crying." The teacher intervenes saying, "He shouldn't be picked up when he cries because he only wants to be the centre of attention. At the beginning he had tantrums, hitting his head on the floor, but now things are better." She then tells Carlo to go play with the others. Still crying, Carlo looks at the other children, but he continues to go towards the observer. He rubs his fists over his eyes, under his nose, along his cheeks and against his ears. He does this repeatedly, sometimes with only one hand, sometimes with both. The observer says, "Carlo is crying and doesn't want to play with the other children." He stares at her, his eyes sad. He moves his fists in front of him and, rotating them, observes his fingers, sticking out first his index finger, then his thumb, and then makes a tight fist. He then puts his hands behind his back, lowers his head, looks at one of the observer's shoes and touches it. He raises his head and sees himself in the mirror in front of him. He looks at the observer again, still holding his hands behind his back. He turns and sees his companions playing. He takes a few hesitant steps and picks up a construction piece and then another and puts them in the observer's hand one at a time. Slowly Carlo goes towards the toy shelf and watches the other children.*

*Franco points the pistol at the observer and even wants to stick it in her mouth, until the observer is forced to say, "You can't do that." Franco stops immediately and runs off with the pistol in his hand.*

*On the other side of the room Elisa is holding the hand of the biggest girl in the class, who has a maternal attitude towards her: she makes Elisa sit down at the table and pretends to feed her.*

*Alice is sitting next to another older girl, but, unlike her sister, she refuses to be picked up or cuddled. Alice goes to the observer and asks what her name is, but just then the older girl puts something on her head. She reacts by tearing apart the object given to her, throwing it on the floor and walks away scowling as she goes. Not looking where she puts her feet, Alice trips over a box of toys; surprised, she cries a little, and the teacher goes to her to see if she is all right.*

*The teacher announces story time and tells the children to put the toys away and each take a chair and form a circle. Alice obeys immediately, followed by the girl that wants to befriend her. Elisa lets her companion treat her as a baby by sitting her down and continuing to cuddle her in a motherly way. Bruno is one of the first to be seated in the circle, and Franco sits next to him with the pistol still in hand. Daniele sits next to Elisa. The teacher has to tell Carlo repeatedly to get a chair, and he finally does, but he sits outside the circle, facing towards the observer* (perhaps searching for a one-to-one relationship that he needs so much). *The younger teacher moves him into the group. Elisa turns around and gives the observer a big smile. Franco and Daniele pretend to shoot at the observer.*

This observation will be discussed in the psychodynamic profiles of the individual sextuplets (see chapter III).

## 13  Leave-taking

The second to last observation (two years and 11 months) takes place in the middle of winter on a foggy and rainy day. There is a depressed atmosphere in the home. The children are still in their pajamas; they are just recovering from the mumps after having been to Rome for a television show.

"Staying home is a disaster!" exclaims the mother, and she adds that next month the helpers stop coming. Solemnly she asks the observer, "So, this is the last time you are coming here?" anticipating by a month the date established for the last observation.

\*\*\*

The last monthly observation (almost three years) takes place around Christmas time and the atmosphere is euphoric. The grandmother at the upstairs window announces the arrival of the observer, who has brought a gift for the sextuplets (six pairs of socks), inciting a small riot as the children want to choose the pair they prefer according to the colour.

The mother calls everyone to order by announcing the morning programme, "Now we'll put on records and then we'll go out in the van."

*When the music begins, the mother starts dancing with Bruno. Franco makes big circles around the armchair to the rhythm of the music. Elisa turns round and round with her arms outstretched, moving her fingers. Carlo slowly calms down from a tantrum, goes back onto the rug and begins to dance; one of his shoes comes off and he takes it to the observer to have it put back on. Alice who is in her mother's arms wants to dance and Bruno moves happily around the room with Franco. Alice lets her head fall back while the mother circles rapidly around in the room. Whenever there is a brief interval between two songs, Franco stops and waits. "There's a march," announces the mother, putting Alice down, and now they all circle around in the room … . "Now let's get in the van … . Grandpa's ready."*

The mother drives the van to the destination chosen by Alice, who wants to see the nativity scene in a nearby church. They stop in front of the church and the children are taken inside. People begin to arrive for the Sunday mass and the group of sextuplets becomes the centre of attention. The priest invites the children to remain for the mass, even though the mother is worried about not being able to control the situation.

Hence the religious ceremony occupies most of the observation at the end of which the mother delegates the grandfather to take the observer back to her car. During the ride the grandfather mentions that he is worried about Carlo who "seems different from the others, and doesn't talk as well as they do".

The observation ends without a real farewell and it is the only time that the mother and the sextuplets do not return home with the observer who feels that she is the one who is left out, and used as a depository for unpleasant and angry feelings. The mother does not say good-bye and, as on other occasions, chooses to be out or busy in order to avoid facing the pain of separation and endings.

## 14   The third year: "Staying at home is a disaster"

As agreed, the 30th observation takes place six months later when the sextuplets are three and a half years old.

The grandmother informs the observer about the children: *they have had an intestinal disturbance, the toilet training has improved, and only Carlo does not use the potty. The news is that they are all going to the seaside for the weekend: they'll leave Friday evening after dinner and return right after dinner on Sunday, when the children are all asleep and ready to be slipped into bed as soon as they get home.*

*When the mother arrives she says that last spring the whole family went to Japan for ten days, sponsored by a Japanese television channel. The trip was very tiring for all of them. Then, at the beginning of June, they spent a week at the beach, guests of a company that manages a vacation village.* "We inaugurated it!"

And that was not all! The mother had also written a book with the help of a journalist to "tell other women about my experience ... . I don't know whether I would advise others to make the same decision I did or not."

*The children look bigger, except for Elisa, who is dressed like a little lady with a coloured skirt, clogs, and a scarf on her head; all the others are wearing shorts. Their clothes are dirty and full of stains, their shoes worn out, their hair uncombed, and their hands dirty.* Well, it is summer and the children stay outside a lot, but it is also the first time the observer sees them looking untidy.

The boys stay mostly with a visiting uncle; the two sisters are together doing girlish games. *Elisa is busy folding a dress and Alice takes hold of a push-chair and declares, "This is for us women ...." Elisa announces, touching her head, that she is Lina (a cousin). Alice then helps her sister squeeze in-between her and the handles of the push-chair (her favourite position) and they walk together [...]. When the mother says to Elisa, "Well, how is my little lady?", Alice goes towards her brothers and grabs a toy out of Bruno's hand; he is offended and begins to cry. The mother says to Alice, "That's enough! Why did you do that?", and the little girl replies proudly, "Because I am me!"*

*Later the conflict between them is repeated when the mother threatens Alice that the strawberries she is eating will give her a bellyache because they are not ripe. Alice replies, "Not true" and continues eating,* manifesting once again her strong and stubborn character trait.

Six months later the 31st and last observation (three years and six months) takes place the day after Christmas. The mother is preparing dinner for 30 people. She says that the children have destroyed the nativity scene under their Christmas tree, and that now they are all going out for a ride in the van with the father.

*The mother turns on the radio. The father is driving; he turns off the radio and invites the children to tell a story. Alice* (who, as usual, takes the lead as the "first-born") *says she is ready, but Bruno wants to be the first. The father decides to let Bruno begin, but the boy remains silent, blocked and looks away with his chin raised. So the father tells his sister to begin, and Alice says, "Once upon a time there was a king ... and they lived happily ever after." Elisa begins with the same words, but the story goes off course as she talks about her fingers and the mother supplies missing words. Daniele talks about an airplane "that flies towards the clouds ... to Japan"* (telling a true story instead of making one up). *The father pays attention to what they all say and makes comments about each story, as if he were the moderator. At this point Bruno begins to tell a story about "pooh-pooh", and laughs. Carlo does not participate; the father tries to get him involved by asking him a few questions, but he does not respond.*

*Bruno moves close to Elisa, who was silent and alone, and continues his story about "pooh-pooh", and they smile together. Then Bruno pulls Elisa's hair, but she ignores him and then she begins a story about "hair pulling". They continue to play and bother each other.* Bruno seems to be making a show of his linguistic abilities, with Elisa's complicity.

*All of a sudden the mother asks what Franco is doing: "He's not sleeping, is he?" Franco pretends to be asleep while Alice looks at him and replies that he is. The mother says, "It's not nap time!" In response to this Franco and Elisa lie down on the floor of the van and with big smiles on their faces close their eyes.* Franco seems to be the central figure of a mischievous trio that has fun teasing their mother-teacher.

*After a brief visit to relatives the group accompanies the observer to her car, at full speed and with loud music from the radio. At a certain point it is the mother who falls asleep with her head leaning against the car window. The father glances at her a few times. As soon as she wakes up she says she could have slept longer and she suggests that the children sing.*

When they arrive at the house they let the observer get out and the mother says: "Call me whenever you want." The observer says good-bye to the children, who are still in the van and staring at her.

The last three observations, done in a one-year period, show the children's development as they grow, their individual temperaments, habits, tastes, reciprocal choices, and how they play, as well as their conflicts and quarrels. The relationships with the parents and grandparents become more clearly delineated. All these aspects will be investigated further in the next chapter.

CHAPTER THREE

# Psychodynamic profiles
# of the individual sextuplets

In this chapter we present six individual psychodynamic profiles,
based principally on the observational material, a brief relational-
neuromotor evaluation (done by a child neuro-psychiatrist,
Adriano Milani Comparetti, when the sextuplets were one and a
half months old), and the observation and findings of the Brunet-
Lezine test (done when they were 14 months and 18 days old). The
profiles describe the evolution and the personality development of
the individual children, allowing the longitudinal development of
each child as foreseen by the Bick method to be perceived.

To facilitate the reader's understanding we have divided the individual profiles into paragraphs that contain significant aspects of the
interactions between the individual child and the family environment, and among the sextuplets. Specific observational sequences
have been chosen to evidence typical behaviors and emerging characteristics that are repeated and evolve over time. In this way the
observational sequences come to represent a verifiable, scientifically
valid narrative of each child's development. As D. Vallino so aptly
states: "The truthfulness of an observation develops over time; it
evidences a characteristic congruity between the sessions and permits one to see the compatibility of the different readings of the

Table 1. Essential data.

| Name | Birth order | Birth weight (grams) | Return home | Observer's perception |
|------|-------------|----------------------|-------------|-----------------------|
| Alice | 1st | 1 500 | 1st | the firstborn |
| Bruno | 2nd | 1 750 | 1st | the solitary child |
| Carlo | 3rd | 1 600 | 5th | the damaged child |
| Daniele | 4th | 1 450 | 2nd | the forgotten child |
| Elisa | 5th | 1 200 | 3rd | Grandma's *pet* |
| Franco | 6th | 1 550 | 2nd/4th | the boy baby |

sequences. One cannot consider the facts observed as understood or interpreted until this characteristic has been achieved" (1996, p. 29).

We also present some of the thoughts and hypotheses discussed during the *Infant Observation* seminars and during our research project.

The table below (table 1) lists essential data that can help the reader to keep in mind and distinguish individually each sextuplet. The names of the children are imaginary and follow an alphabetical order for the same purpose. In addition to some basic information (birth weight, birth order, order of the children's move from hospital to go home following their births), the table includes a very brief description of the observer's perception of each child at the end of the infant observation period.

## Alice: The firstborn

Alice was the first to be born. Her birth weight was 1500 grams, and she weighed 3080 grams when she was taken home from the hospital.

Neuromotor-relational evaluation (one and a half months): "Good attention to environmental stimuli and good postural control; movements better than those of her siblings."

### First impressions

Alice seems older than her siblings, both in her behaviour and in terms of how she is treated. *As soon as the mother hears her voice coming from the bedroom, she runs to get her, and shows her to the observer. She points out how the baby holds her arms flexed outwards away from her body,* as if she were making space for herself (six and a half months).

*The mother says that Alice is the only one* [of the six] *who doesn't smile much, she is a serious baby and an aunt confirms this opinion when she says that Alice is very determined: "When she wants something, only that will do! She is just like her mother when she was little"* (nine and a half months).

*As soon as she is awake, Alice immediately stands up. She holds onto the side of the cot and looks at the grandmother and the observer without smiling. Then she kneels, hiding her face as if she wants to play peek-a-boo, but she continues to sulk* (11 months).

*This little girl does not seek hugs from anyone; she sucks her thumb but does not want a dummy. Once she sucked her thumb with such great satisfaction that she undid a bow tied to the cot and almost swallowed it. [...] Bruno and Franco greet the observer (who just arrived) with big smiles, but Alice doesn't seem to see her and continues sucking her thumb enthusiastically* (seven and a half months).

The mother often tries to engage her in playing a game where they take turns sticking out their tongues (six and a half months). Sometimes she encourages the child to send kisses.

During the two observations (seven and eight months) the mother and the children are guests in the lovely garden of a distinguished neighbour; the gentleman appears to want to establish a special relationship with Alice, paying her compliments, holding her, and teasing that she wants to stay with him only when she chooses. He nicknames her Pandora, the mythical personage who by opening her box released all the ills known to mankind.

## Alice's "progress"

She is the first of the sextuplets to walk, at 12½ months.

The mother states that Alice does not want to eat what the other sextuplets eat (14 months). The grandmother says that she already wants to eat with the grown-ups and that she is the one who establishes the rhythm of the meals, by opening and closing her mouth as she wishes (13 months).

She is the only one of the sextuplets to welcome in the first new year with her parents and grandparents, having awakened around midnight.

At 18 months Alice has the privilege of being the only one to go to the seaside with the grandparents, a privilege that the mother soon recognizes as dangerous: *"She had become used to being alone, and we* can't allow that" (18½ months). She does not have trouble going to sleep and does not wake in the night.

The grandmother reports that Alice is the only one to use the potty, "She sits on the throne surrounded by all the others" (two years and nine months).

### The relationship with the father

The father and Alice have a special relationship: she seeks him out and he reciprocates. One gets the impression that a triad is taking shape: mother-father-daughter. *The father leans over towards Alice and she opens her arms and stretches her legs. She grabs her father's nose, but suddenly he moves away because she has scratched him. He then offers her a necklace with shiny dangles that Alice plays with happily* (eight and a half months).

*As soon as the father enters the living room Alice jumps with joy. He leans over and kisses her on the forehead, then gives her a pat on the head and says "Snuggle-bug"* (10½ months).

The grandmother says: "*Alice really likes her father! And he has a weak spot for her* (11 months). And again a month later: "*… What a joy it is for this little girl when her father comes home!*"

*When Alice discovers that her father is in the bedroom, she trots off to find him, with all the other sextuplets trailing behind. They wait outside the door. Then the others seem to lose interest and disappear and Alice remains alone with her father* (13½ months).

In another observation *the father arrives and the children all run to him yelling: "Daddy, Daddy." He greets them one by one. Then they all go back to their play, except for Alice who stays next to him and he leans over, gives her a hug and whispers something in her ear* (21 months).

### Play

Through play Alice expresses her world of fantasy in which she seems to show off and imitate grown-ups.

*When the grandmother offers the observer coffee, Alice immediately offers her own piece of bread […]. She tries to open a cabinet in the kitchen, tearing away a piece of tape that has been used to keep it closed. The child ignores the grandmother's warning not to do it and pulls the tape with all her strength, banging her feet on the floor. The grandmother insists on her rules, pulls the girl's hands away and closes the door with the tape. Alice then throws herself down on the floor and cries in despair while kicking and rolling her body back and forth. The grandmother calls the helper and says that Alice needs to be changed because she has done a pooh-pooh. "She did so much!" comments the helper, after cleaning her with wet cotton. Alice complains for a little longer, then remains silent for a moment while she tries to touch herself between her legs* (16½ months).

The adults treat her as if she were older. For example: *the grand-mother tells Alice to go and see if Daniele is awake* (18 months).

*The mother tells her to pretend to telephone Daddy [...]. Then, when mother announces that lunch is ready, Alice immediately begins to gather up the toys and put them in the playpen. The mother says:"Good girl! It's always you and I who do this job, my big girl!" Alice is so pleased and starts to run about until she is out of breath. [...] Afterwards the mother tells her to smell her sister to find out if she has done a pooh-pooh* (22 months).

*The mother shows her new tennis shoes to Alice, who immediately shows her own saying "new shoes". The mother* (in competition with her daughter) *then explains that her shoes are new, but that Alice's are not* (22 months).

*Alice takes a ride on the tricycle. She manages to go up a step, but has difficulty going down and says to herself, "Be careful of the step"* (28½ months).

*After the helper leaves, the grandmother gets angry because the children won't obey her. Alice quickly lines up the folding chairs, a task usually done by the helper* (two years and seven months).

## The relationship between the two sisters

Some of the observations suggest a particular pattern in the rela-tionship between Alice and Elisa, one in which the former takes the initiative and the latter follows suit.

*Alice and Elisa circle round the armchair where the observer is sitting, each holding a scarf. Elisa sees another scarf on the floor; she drops the one she already has and picks up the new one. Alice grabs it out of her hand quickly and moves backwards holding it close. Elisa yells and calls the helper. Alice notices that the observer is watching the scene and assumes an air of importance. She leans on the arm of the observer's chair and gently touches her necklace saying "little balls", and then walks with a swaggering gait toward the helper* (25½ months).

*The helper and Elisa remount the pieces of a toy mill that fell while the little girl was carrying them. Alice notices the toy and attempts to grab it away from her sister* (two years and four months).

In another observation *Elisa copies her sister who is putting the children's chairs in place. When Alice changes her mind and wants to play with the puppet theatre, Elisa immediately begins to tidy up to make space for the new game, as if she were Alice's assistant* (two years and six months).

### The Brunet-Lezine test (14 months, 12 days)

The mother chooses Alice to be the second child to be tested, and before the test begins she asks for a pillow because, she says, the table is too high for the little girl. The father hands the pillow to the mother as the little girl watches them attentively (see *His Majesty the Child*, Freud, 1914).

Throughout the trials the little girl "chatters" as if she were imitating the examiner or the mother. After the block trial, which she does well, while the examiner is writing her notes, the mother puts her face next to her daughter's, takes her hands in her own and places them over her eyes. Then the mother draws her hands away saying "peek-a-boo", as if she, too, wanted to be an examiner and give her child a test. During the second trial Alice is so absorbed playing with the blocks that the examiner, almost as if she felt intimidated, says she is sorry to have to take them away. All in all the child does the test well. During the last trial she holds the pencil "correctly, just like an adult", as the examiner writes in her notes. At the end of the test the mother has difficulty taking Alice away because she holds on to the table as if she did not want to leave.

### At the nursery school (two years, nine months, 12 days)

Alice behaves like an independent, self-sufficient little girl. She plays well alone, and refuses to play with an older girl who wants her to play the part of a little girl. In order to defend her brother Daniele she vents her aggressiveness by hitting a little boy, chosen at random. Then at a certain point, using a tone of authority like a teacher doing roll-call, she asks the observer what her name is.

*Personality traits and relational characteristics*

From the very first observation we note that Alice receives a lot of attention from her mother, who seems to assign her the role of "best student". The little girl responds by showing good psycho-motor development and often being the first of the sextuplets to reach certain developmental milestones. The fact that she was the first to be born and the first (with Bruno) to go home from the hospital probably contributed to the family's image of her as the "first" or "eldest" child.

Alice experiences the mother's perceptions and attributions regarding her in an ego-synchronic way, giving her mother satisfaction and her mother, in turn, seems to identify with her narcissistically.

Alice also has a special relationship with her father. This seems to have contributed to the formation of a strong sense of self-esteem and to be the basis for her female narcissism, whereas the strong identification with the mother may have made it more difficult for her to express Oedipal rivalry with her mother.

Alice behaves as if she were older than her siblings; she likes to command them and tends to treat them as if she were an adult who can impose her ideas upon others; she appears to identify more with a mother figure and very little with her siblings.

She bears some resemblance to Ruth, a little girl described in Anna Freud and Sophie Dann's study (1951) of a group of orphaned children. In the group, Ruth was the only child who had a relationship with the mother in the first months after birth. And for that reason she would seek out an adult figure and was less integrated in the group.

This is a well known study of a group of six orphans who were together for almost three years during WWII, beginning from when they were between six and 12 months old, in the facility for orphans run by the prisoners in the Theresienstadt concentration camp. After the war the children were transferred to a special home in England. The authors of the study observed that there was a primary attachment between the six children that could not be substituted by any adult attachment and that this rather unusual collaborative behaviour was due to the total absence of an adult to whom they could become attached during early infancy.

## Bruno: The solitary child

Bruno was the second to be born; his birth weight was 1750 grams and when he was taken home he weighed 3760 grams.

Neuromotor-relational evaluation (one and a half months): "The child is rather slow and not very efficient in his postural motor response, but he shows attention to his surroundings. Prognosis reserved; he will need to be re-evaluated."

### First impressions

This healthy, sweet-looking child has a delicate, docile character. In the first observation *he is sleeping on his belly with his legs stretched out, and when his mother calls him he turns immediately towards her with a big smile and gurgles as if he were replying.*

From the very beginning the mother encourages him to interact with her, as if she had expectations regarding his verbal and intellectual capabilities.

*Bruno, looking at the mother, holds the dummy in his hand near his mouth and gurgles* (seven and a half months).

*Bruno and the grandmother are conversing: he is saying "Da-Da" and the mother says he speaks German. [...] As soon as the mother returns home, Bruno begins to trill his lips going "Brrrr", spitting out saliva and smiling as if he wanted to talk. The mother says that until a month ago he didn't say anything at all, adding that he still can't stand up* (nine and a half months).

According to the mother he is aware of what people are doing. The observer notices that he often follows his mother's movements with his eyes (13½ months).

*As soon as the mother begins to prepare to go out Bruno follows her every movement attentively, watching her until she has gone out of the door* (11 months).

*Bruno never takes his eyes off his mother as she looks for her handbag before going out shopping* (15 months).

*After the mother has left the house, the grandmother asks the children where she is and Bruno stares at the door for a long time* (16 months).

*Bruno is the only one who is aware of the bell that indicates the mother has returned, and he announces it to the group: "Mamma, Mamma". Later he tries to mess up the mother's hair, but she ignores him because she is too busy with the other children. [...] Bruno brushes his hand against one of the observer's shoes to get her attention. He then touches the shoe, pronounces the word shoe, and disappears behind the armchair. When he comes out on the other side there is a sound of music and the helper says, "Bravo. Bruno has put on a record ... ."* The other children all say, "Di-co, di-co" (for the Italian word *"disco"* which means record), *while Bruno sings softly, concentrating on the words of the song* (25 months).

The mother often and unexpectedly asks him to give her a kiss (12th, 13th, 17th observations).

*Motor difficulties*

Bruno is not very agile or physically active. He appears to be most sensitive to visual and auditory stimuli. Although he was the first of the sextuplets to sit up, he was one of the last to walk. The mother reports that he walked all of a sudden, but skipped all the intermediate phases like crawling. Perhaps this is related to a difficulty about separating from his mother.

*When he was nine and a half months old he falls backwards, hitting his head on the floor, and cries very hard. The mother picks him up and bounces him on her knees. Bruno laughs contentedly, but instead of looking at her he keeps his head turned away as if he were unhappy with her ...* (nine and a half months).

At 12½ months Bruno suffers a more serious head trauma when he falls backwards a second time, hitting his head on the floor so hard that he is taken to the hospital emergency room. The parents are very worried and the doctor advises close supervision for a month. The mother reports that after the last injury Bruno had almost forgotten how to walk and the father jokingly calls him "broken head" (14 months).

*The children are with the grandmother and the helper in the yard at the country house. The mother is out. The helper, tired after playing for a long time with the children, proposes that they all sit down. Bruno finds a small folding chair that the helper opens up for him. While Bruno sits down in front of the helper, she gets up to get Carlo who is "bothering grandmother". When she picks up Carlo, taking him into her arms, Bruno falls from his chair and cries.* Perhaps this was an awkward and indirect way of expressing jealousy and disappointment (two years and four months).

## Play

Bruno prefers to play alone; he appears very concentrated on what he is doing and tends to isolate himself from the other sextuplets. His interests are sedentary: he likes to listen to records or music on the radio. He is above all very attentive to the mother's whereabouts.

*Bruno comes in and looks towards the light and says, "Oh-oh". "It's the light," responds the mother, adding that he always notices the light, and Bruno repeats, "Oh-oh"* (15 months).

*The mother points out the drawing of a bell tower that goes ding-dong, and Bruno responds pointing at the light, saying "Uce-uce",* referring to the Italian word *"luce"* which means light. *As soon as he is on his feet after being changed, Bruno turns towards the light, points at it, and smiles* (18 months).

*When the observer arrives Bruno is in the middle of the living room playing by himself and murmuring almost imperceptibly. The mother says, with evident satisfaction, that Bruno has discovered that the two loud-speakers emit different sounds because once during an advertisement he noticed that vocal music came from one and background music from the other* (23 months).

*The mother gets out of the van and Bruno notices that the light over the door has remained lit. He brings it to the attention of the helper who discovers that the door has not been closed.* (two years and two months).

Bruno likes to play girl-type games, like playing "ladies" with Alice.

*The grandmother welcomes the observer and invites her into the kitchen. She says that the mother is at the new house cleaning it up for when they move in, and that they are planning to take the children to the seaside for the weekend. Alice is looking at a magazine and Bruno has the small espresso coffee pot in his hands and pretends to drink from the spout [...]. The helper arrives and suggests he give Alice some coffee. Bruno, showing off, stands up and drinks from the spout. Alice runs towards him and Bruno says: "Mrs. Alice, come and have some coffee." The helper gives them a plastic cup [...]. Afterwards, Bruno pretends to pour coffee on the other sister's head; the helper tells him not to because Elisa's hair would get dirty and she suggests that, instead, he pretends to be a hairdresser* (two years and four months).

During the first year he was often paired with Elisa in the play-pen (eight and a half months) or the pram (12½ months). They were also in the same class at nursery school. Their responses in adolescence to the socio-relational questionnaire (part b, past), reveal a feeling of affinity between brother and sister (see chapter IV, paragraph 2).

He does not take any initiative in establishing social relationships, neither with his brothers and sisters nor with other adults, except for the mother who is the only person about whom he seems to care and with whom he wants to be. He is possessive of her and jealous of her relationships with the other sextuplets.

*Temperamental behaviour*

Bruno is touchy and moody.

The mother says that he *smiles a lot, sleeps a lot, and cries a lot*. The observer notes that when he cries he expresses sadness and discomfort, rather than anger (seven and a half months).

*Bruno is listening to music on the radio and Franco grabs a toy out of Carlo's hand. The father is watching, he wiggles his finger and says "No" in a calm, firm voice and explains that this is not the way to act. Then Bruno goes over to Carlo and tries to take the toy away from him; again the father says a solemn "No". All of a sudden Bruno lies down on the marble floor, his head pointing away from the father, and he has an almost offended air. When the father tells him to get up, Bruno looks sulky, withdraws further, and remains immobile* (24 months).

According to the mother Bruno *is the perfect child at school: he listens, understands, and does everything well. He is happy there, but when he comes home he is agitated and causes trouble* (two years and seven months).

*The grandmother tells Bruno and Elisa to show the observer their bedroom. Elisa responds as if she had some doubts about complying. Bruno, however, starts off and the grandmother says: "OK, take the lady's hand." Bruno refuses to do so, but his more outgoing sister willingly takes the observer's hand. Bruno turns on the light at the bottom of the stairs and the children go up without holding the railing. When they arrive at the top Bruno runs enthusiastically towards the bedroom and throws himself on a bed exclaiming, "This is Bruno's." The grandmother corrects him: "No, that's Franco's," and then closes the window to keep the flies out. Bruno sees a bottle on a dresser and says "Perfume". A little later when the children go back down the stairs, Bruno goes down cautiously, leaning slightly against the wall while Elisa runs down quickly, so much so that the grandmother tells her to go slower* (two years and seven months).

### Brunet-Lezine test (14 months, 18 days)

Bruno was the only one of the sextuplets to refuse to do the test. The mother had Elisa take his place and he was rescheduled to last place. When he did do the test, he performed well and quickly in all the trials.

The mother says that he is "very capable, and he can even build a tower with five blocks". In fact, as soon as the examiner gives him the blocks, Bruno begins to build a tower, with two and then three blocks. The examiner notes that "he is very careful and delicate in his movements". Afterwards, Bruno picks up the cup and then puts it upside down on the table and places blocks on it, making another tower. At this point the mother, preceding the examiner, shows him how to put the blocks into the cup and he does it. The mother says, "Now it will be hard to take them away from him." Then Bruno dumps them all into her lap. He performs the spoon trial correctly and then puts the spoon into his mouth. He also does the bottle and tablet trial well, and when he has taken the tablet out of the bottle he turns towards his mother and offers it to her. The mother opens her mouth and takes it. Then Bruno tries to find it, putting his hand in her mouth. He does the bell trial well. The mother then takes the initiative again: noticing that Bruno is attracted by a red block on the floor, she requests that the napkin trial be done with that block instead of with the bell. Bruno manages to put the round object into the hole on the board all by himself. He scribbles right away with the pencil, and then begins to "talk" to it. At the end the examiner takes note that "he has long conversations composed of many different sounds".

### At the nursery school (two years, nine months, 12 days)

Bruno stays by himself, although he understands and pays careful attention to what is going on around him, but without taking part. He seems to keep a check from afar on what is happening. When the teacher asks the children if anyone has seen a small piece of a toy that is part of a game she is putting away, Bruno who has it in his hand looks at it but he does not give it to her. This is a rather ambiguous behaviour for such an intelligent child that leaves some doubt about his true intentions.

*Personality traits and relational characteristics*

This child appears to be placid and tranquil; he is very attentive and reflective. His remarkable capacity to concentrate his attention for long periods of time are in tune with the mother's expectations. Bruno shows particular sensitivity to visual and auditory stimuli. He is attracted to and fascinated by his mother: when she is present, he never takes his eyes off her, as if he lived in her shadow.

His clumsiness, evidenced by some bad falls, seems to be due more to the fear of separation from the mother and losing a place in her mind than to any specific motorial difficulties. This strong fusional need is not actively pursued, but is expressed by his moody behaviour.

Bruno does not have frequent dealings with his brothers; he seems to have more affinity with his sisters. He is often separate from the rest of the sextuplet group, absorbed in solitary, sedentary play. He is rarely openly aggressive, except with Carlo. In moments of conflict with his siblings he usually freezes: he does not react directly by getting angry or hitting someone, but remains immobile and tense as if he were offended.

## Carlo: The damaged child

Carlo was ·the third sextuplet to be born; his birth weight was 1600 grams and he weighed 3080 grams when he was taken home. He had been operated on for inguinal hernia before being sent home from the hospital.

Neuromotor-relational evaluation (one and a half months): "It is impossible to say whether psychomotor functions are normal at this time", because he is recovering from surgery.

*First impressions*

From the first observation Carlo appears to be a lazy, despondent baby, slow in his movements and uninterested in his surroundings.

*When he has just woken and the mother takes him into her arms, Carlo leans his head on her shoulder holding his fists tightly against his body. "He's bashful!" exclaims the mother.*

He is the only one of the sextuplets whom the mother gives the observer to hold, as if he needed more care than the others. She points out the particular shape of the child's head, "*long and narrow, very probably due to the fact that they were so cramped in the womb*" (a maternal fantasy of foetal suffering?).

*Carlo falls backwards and cries but doesn't try to get up. The mother goes to him and puts him on his feet saying, "You have a heavy bottom." She holds his hands and helps him move backwards and forwards. He allows her to cuddle him, but he keeps his head lowered, practically between his shoulders. "He is the slowest," says the mother* (nine and a half months).

*Carlo enters the living room, sits down in a corner and sucks his thumb. He doesn't look at anyone, he is silent, and he seems to move about without any precise destination [...]. Sitting in the play-pen alone, with a dummy in his mouth, he leans to one side with his head buckled over. His movements are awkward and uncoordinated [...]. The mother snaps her fingers near his ear, saying his name, but he does not react, and the father says that he is afraid that the child may be deaf* (10½ months).

*The mother leans down towards Carlo in the baby-walker and shows him the charms on her necklace. As soon as she has his attention she hides the charms under her sweater and waits for his reaction; his attention stays on the movement of her hands rather than the charms. "He doesn't understand," she deduces, and tries the same thing with Elisa who immediately looks for the charms* (12½ months).

The mother worries that he is not receiving enough stimulation.

*The grandmother calls him "Sitting Bull"* (16 months).

*The mother reports that he has quite a few teeth, but he doesn't chew meat* (17 months).

At 18 months, he is the last of the six to learn to walk.

*The father is with the children as they go down the stairs. Carlo goes down sitting on his bottom, staying behind the rest [...].*

*The grandmother is changing Carlo's nappy and he fusses and grabs the edge of his trousers. The grandmother explains, "He doesn't want to see his knees: it's amazing how modest he is!" And she says to the child, "What can grandma do? We need a lot of patience with you." Later Carlo pulls Elisa's hair very hard, and she cries and runs to the grandmother who says, "Carlo is a real handful"* (two years and three months).

*"Poor thing, he'd like to do what the others do, but he just isn't able,"* says the grandmother (two years and five months).

### Relationship with the other sextuplets

He does not relate much to the other sextuplets, except to be a nuisance. He treats them as if they were a bothersome burden and hits them unexpectedly. None of them wants to play with him. Sometimes he is overcome by his siblings who take toys away from him and do things faster. There is evident mutual rejection.

*The mother brings a lot of toys into the room, giving something to each of the children, and then gets ready to go out. She puts her sunglasses on Alice, who shows off proudly. Carlo is sitting with his legs astraddle and whimpers. Bruno watches his mother as she leaves, and then, seeing the sunglasses that his sister has put down, he picks them up. Carlo crawls over and grabs the sunglasses, insisting on having them. Bruno tries to resist and then crying gives them up; he looks at the observer and then at the light on above his head, and says, "Oo-oo"* (15 months).

While driving the van, with all the children in the back, the mother talks with the observer, looking at her in the rearview mirror, and says: *"It's hard to understand Carlo. He has so many tantrums. We know what the others want, but not him; with him it's trial and error." Anyhow, he understands when I say we're going out. Could he be autistic? [...] When the mother suddenly stops the van, opens the door and gets out, Carlo throws a jacket on Elisa's head; she rebels, but he continues, finding it more and more amusing* (two years and two months).

*Someone is crying on the terrace, and Franco comes in touching his head. "What's the matter?" the grandmother asks, adding, "Carlo hit you!" [...] All of a sudden Carlo pulls Elisa's hair; she cries, out of pain and indignation and runs to the grandmother who gives her a pat on the head while scolding: "Carlo, you mustn't do that!"* (two years and three months).

*The mother tells Bruno and Franco to give each other a kiss, and they do so, giving each other a pat on the head, also. They seem amused. After, the mother tells Franco to do the same with Carlo, but Franco shakes his head.*

Bruno teases Carlo about nursery school, saying that he cries and that "He's dumb" (two years and 9 months).

*Temper tantrums*

Temper tantrums refer to "manifestations of acute anxiety so often seen in children between one and five years … (when the child is refused something he wants or when he feels forced to accept something he doesn't want). Tantrums are deaf to the voice of reason or command and almost inaccessible to external influence" (Susan Iaacs, 1946, p. 129).

Carlo has frequent temper tantrums and hits his head anywhere and everywhere when he is at the height of his rage, but shows no signs of pain.

*After the walk the children go into the house and Carlo is put down. All of a sudden he begins to cry, lies down, pulls his hair, and hits his head on the marble floor, and finally, taking one of his shoes in his teeth, he pulls with all his might. The mother offers him a piece of apple, and he takes it. He stands up and goes to a low cabinet in the kitchen; the helper says "No" and takes him away. Carlo then has another tantrum* (18 months).

*The mother calls the sextuplets and says, "Let's go outside." They all follow her except Carlo who has to be picked up and carried. As soon as they are in the garden the mother suggests they play merry-go-round. Carlo cries and wants to be picked up again. The mother says that he was sick for the four days that they (the parents) were at the beach* (19 months).

*The father walks with some of the children, Alice runs back and forth, and the mother is with Carlo who walks slower than the others. The mother is amazed that he isn't crying—which is "so normal for him". Then without warning he begins to cry: first he stamps his feet, then he throws himself belly down on the ground and has a "typical tantrum". The father calls him, then tells Franco to help him. Franco runs to him, falls and then he cries, too* (two years and three months).

*Brunet-Lezine test (14 months, 18 days)*

The mother succeeds in squeezing Carlo into the morning session (as if she wanted to get his test over with), with the excuse that "There's still some time before lunch". She tells the examiner that he is "different" from the other children.

In the first trial Carlo does not pick up the blocks. In the second he looks at the examiner "with a tense expression and remains immobile". The examiner encourages him, smiles, does peek-a-boo, smiles again, calls his name. Carlo begins to cry and looks for the mother, who leans him against her and consoles him saying "Mummy's here." After the napkin trial, in which he manages to discover the bell, he begins to cry again and the mother says, "He makes me suffer." Carlo does not watch as the examiner shows him how to put the round piece into the board and starts to cry.

At a certain point the father announces a phone call for the mother, who gets up leaving the child on the floor with the examiner. He stares at the table leg without responding to the examiner's solicitations. When the mother comes back, the examiner remembers that they have not done the trial with the tablet in the bottle but that trial is also not successful because Carlo looks only at the bottle and ignores the tablet.

The test evidences that Carlo has a developmental problem: the results obtained cannot be codified. The mother says sadly: "He didn't do anything."

### At the nursery school (two years, nine months, 12 days)

Carlo seems disoriented and, as during the test, cries continually. He isolates himself from his siblings and from the other children. The teachers have instructions not to pick him up. He seems to respond to the attention of the observer who, without going beyond her task, verbalizes out loud what is happening, "Carlo is crying". After this Carlo begins to make contact with her, looking at her sadly while trying to make a vague proposal to play. He shows an absolute need for a one-to-one relationship with an adult figure.

### Personality traits and relational characteristics

Carlo's psycho-motor development is different from that of the other sextuplets. The mother thinks that he suffered before birth "because he was too cramped and uncomfortable in the womb" (see chapter II, paragraph 4). He has little response to environmental stimuli: he does not participate in group activities, and he shows no interest in any of his siblings and does not seek out adults. He cries often and avoids eye contact with others. He expresses himself prevalently through violent tantrums, which calls to mind the primitive defence called reversal in which the child's aggressiveness is turned toward himself (Fraiberg, 1981).

Carlo seems to be the only sextuplet who has a special need for personalized care. His request for a one-to-one relationship with the mother, albeit normal, is in fact impossible to realize. Even at school he is systematically frustrated because the teachers follow the mother's instructions to avoid holding him in their arms for any length of time.

The mother states openly that she does not understand him and adds that the other sextuplets do not play with him. Even the other relatives say that Carlo has a harder time than his brothers and sisters. Sometimes the mother does not respond to his signs of discomfort: she appears to be blind to his needs. Perhaps it is too painful for her to accept the role of a supportive teacher for a mentally challenging pupil.

## Daniele: The forgotten child

Daniele is the fourth baby to be born. He weighed 1450 grams at birth and 2870 when taken home. He underwent emergency surgery for an inguinal hernia a few days before the neurological examination.

Neuromotor-relational evaluation (one and a half months): "Habitual position with head rotated towards the right (see Armstrong). We recommend subjecting him to stimuli from the other side [...]. He follows recognizably, but dully with his eyes. Prognosis of normality to be verified through systematic controls."

### First impressions

Daniele is the only one of the sextuplets whom the mother does not present to the observer and about whom she makes no personalized comments nor indications of familial resemblance. For a long time the observer has difficulty in individuating him among the sextuplets and tends to confuse him with Franco, the brother with whom he most often plays.

Daniele is usually left on his own until he manifests some particular physical need, such as wanting to eat or go to sleep or be changed. In fact, during the first observation the only interaction between the mother and Daniele is when she changes his nappy.

The mother calls him the "dummy maniac" because Daniele almost always has a dummy in his mouth and sometimes he even holds another in his hand, perhaps a sort of guarantee of continuous gratification (2nd, 3rd, 4th, 6th, 12th and 18th observations).

*Daniele lets Franco hit him until the dummy falls out of his mouth. At that point he starts to cry in anger, but he accepts being hit again as soon as he has recovered the pacifier* (24 months).

*Daniele takes the dummy out of his mouth to eat but as soon as he finishes his food he pops it back in* (two years and six months).

Daniele does not seem to take much notice of the observer: he rarely looks or smiles at her. One of the few times that he is not running all over the place, the observer is able to take a good look at him, and she describes him as having "mischievously slanted eyes, a round nose, and a cheerful smile" that resembles the face of a clown (11½ months).

## Hyperactivity

Right from the beginning it is easy to see that Daniele relishes physical movement. He shows precocious motor development and is a very active, excitable child, constantly moving about except when he collapses from fatigue. In fact he was absent from the 4th and 5th observations (nine and a half and 10½ months) because he was so sleepy that he had to be put to bed at the beginning of the observation.

He is the first of the sextuplets to stand up, but he walks only when holding on to something. He tends to crawl beyond the living room rug, the children's play area.

*Daniele climbs quickly up the net of the play-pen and the grandmother informs the observer that "A few days ago he got out, but he didn't cry. How did he manage not to get hurt?"* (nine and a half months).

*He climbs up the side of the cot like a monkey, and lays there in a horizontal position, apparently happy and comfortable* (23 months).

Daniele sometimes puts himself in risky situations.

*He leans dangerously over the edge of the kitchen table* (23 months).

*The mother reports that one morning Daniele leaned far out of the bedroom window, upstairs, to watch his father take the car out of the garage, asking him calmly: "Are you going to work, Daddy?" "What a fright we had!" she comments* (two years and five months).

*While the mother is changing him, she asks: "Where's Daddy?" Daniele looks towards the picture on the wall behind the changing table, repeating the word "Daddy". Then, as soon as he is undressed, he touches his genitals with his hands* (18 months).

*After changing Franco, the mother sniffs Daniele and decides to change him even though he is not dirty. He touches his genitals as soon as he is undressed; the mother takes his penis in her hand and asks him where it is. He has an erection and looks intensely at the mother's face, and she begins to wash him, applies some cream to his genitals, and puts his nappy on. Then she dresses him quickly and puts him down on the floor* (23 months).

## Daring Daniele

He is hyperactive, somewhat of a bully, aimless in play and indifferent towards others.

*Daniele is in the play-pen with Alice. They are playing together, moving their legs so that their feet touch, and gurgling; every once in a while they throw toys around. All of a sudden Daniele notices his brothers moving around in a baby-walker outside the play-pen. He immediately stands up and tries to climb up the netting to get out. He cries a bit, then, angry and frustrated, goes back down the netting and gives his sister a push. She moves over to make room for him, but he pushes her again, even butting her with his head* (12½ months).

*Daniele notices that Franco and Alice have both received a piece of bread from the grandmother who is preparing the meal. Bruno goes to the kitchen, too, and gets a piece. Daniele goes up to Bruno and tries to take his piece of bread away from him. Bruno objects but can't defend himself from the attack* (15 months).

*Daniele goes into the living room holding a plastic bottle with two spoons inside. He shakes the bottle and listens to the noise it makes, then tries to take the spoons out, but doesn't succeed. Franco goes by and grabs the bottle away from him. Daniele protests, throws himself down on the floor and yells with rage. The helper gives him a dummy and he gets up and runs off […]. Alice picks up two wooden blocks, then goes near the grandmother and hits them together. She then gives them to another little girl who is visiting. Franco likes this game: he gets two blocks for himself and wanders around the room hitting them together. Daniele does the same thing, wandering around Bruno and Carlo who remain sitting where they were. All of a sudden Daniele hits Bruno on the head with his blocks.*

*The grandmother scolds him severely, but he ignores her and goes towards the entrance continuing to hit the blocks together* (16 months).

*Daniele grabs a piece of bread out of Carlo's hand [...] and the mother says that he once put a bucket on his head, making his brothers and sisters laugh:* the clown! (19 months).

He has the same behaviour with the father. *As soon as they return from a ride the father helps the children get out of the van. Franco is trying to climb up the step towards the front door and Daniele wants to do what his brother is doing. The father tells him not to do it and wiggles his finger in a "no" sign right in front of his face. Daniele listens, hesitates for a moment, then turns around and takes off towards the step. The father repeats the gesture more firmly. Daniele stops, looks at his father, imitates his gesture with his finger, and then goes off in the opposite direction* (14 months).

## Misunderstandings

Throughout the three year period of observations there are frequent episodes in which the adults do not seem to understand Daniele's needs and behaviour. They either ignore him or forget that he is present.

*Daniele emits brief squeals of anger and the father incites his brother, Franco, who is in the play-pen with him, saying: "Get him, get him, Franco"* (eight and a half months).

*Suddenly Daniele cries because one of his hands is caught in the wheel of the baby-walker. The mother picks him up saying, "I knew this would happen!"* as if she were blaming him instead of consoling him (12½ months).

*Franco grabs a toy away from Daniele who throws himself down on the floor crying, desolated. The helper gives him a dummy to console him* (16 months).

*All at once Daniele falls against Alice, who becomes furious and yells, kicks, and pulls his hair. The mother runs over, releases Alice's grip from his hair saying, "You mustn't pull hair." Then she turns to Daniele and giving him a pat on the head says, "You must have taken a toy away from her"* implying that it was probably his own fault (19 months).

*Daniele begins to yell because his brother has grabbed something away from him, and the father gives him some water to drink* (21 months).

*Daniele wants to take a pair of socks from a package that the mother is showing the observer. He throws himself down on the floor kicking and yelling. The mother quickly reorders the socks in the box after showing him a pair to distract him* (two years and 10 months).

### Brunet-Lezine test (14 months, 18 days)

Daniele is the third of the sextuplets to do the test. He practically starts by himself by throwing all three blocks on the floor until the examiner shows him how to build a tower. When the blocks are put back on the table, he busily moves them back and forth and then thrusts one threateningly near the examiners face; then he builds a tower. In the second trial, and all the subsequent ones, he moves a lot, almost frenetically and chaotically, while the mother seems distracted and lost in her thoughts. She holds the child tightly with her hands around his waist but remains silent and seems unaware of what is going on. In the bottle and tablet trial Daniele does not put the tablet into the bottle; instead, he puts the bottle in his mouth and sucks on it. In the last trial he immediately puts the pencil into his mouth and the examiner says, "You like sucking, don't you?" and shows him how to use it. Daniele looks at her, picks up another pencil and scribbles on a piece of paper, continuing to suck on the first one. In the shape table trial, after having thrown the round piece on the floor a few times he takes it and puts it in the correct hole, takes it out and then puts it in again, without any explanations from anyone. The father comes in to get him and Daniele waves goodbye. When the father puts him down on his feet, he lies down on the floor and lets himself be pulled away by his legs. This test experience evidences that Daniele is hyperactive and generally uncooperative.

### At the nursery school (two years, nine months, 12 days)

Daniele does not stand out among the children and does not seek relationships with anyone—his siblings, the other children, or the teachers. Only in the episode when he bumps into another little boy is he noticed by both the observer and Alice, and the latter goes to his defence. The only time he plays with another child is when at the very end of the observation he and Franco use the pistol pretending to shoot at the observer.

*Personality traits and relational characteristics*

Daniele is rarely seen or heard. His behaviour is characterized by excitability and impulsiveness; he is unable to modulate his physical activity and oscillates between frenetic movement and sudden sleepiness. Palacio-Espasa suggests (1999) that this oscillating behaviour in babies is characteristic of a mood disorder.

He likes strong sensorial stimulation and uses the dummy spasmodically, which seems to interfere with his developing verbal communication. Unable to develop adequate internal resources, Daniele depends above all on his physical capacities, and concrete bodily experience of the self. This suggests the formation of a second skin, described by Esther Bick (1968).

He appears to be inattentive and reckless and has a detached indifferent attitude towards others, whom he considers more as objects than persons. The relationship between the mother and Daniele suggests a lack of a secure attachment that could probably lead to an emotional deficit in Daniele.

## Elisa: Grandma's "pet"

Elisa was the fourth to be born; her birth weight was 1200 grams, and she left the hospital weighing 2590 grams.

Neuromotor-relational evaluation (one and a half months): "Scarce postural control of her head and forward movement; very torpid response to stimuli, but attentive to her surroundings [...]. Favourable prognosis to be confirmed in subsequent controls."

*First impressions*

In the first observation Elisa is in a baby carriage in the living room, separated from the rest of the group, and "is playing tranquilly with a rubber deer". The grandmother introduces her as "the little one" whom she usually takes care of, implying that the mother has given her the maternal role in regard to this child from the outset. The grandmother is the one who usually feeds Elisa. Later on, when the child goes to nursery school, the grandmother blames an episode of intestinal disturbance on the school food, convinced that it cannot be the food she has prepared and given her.

*The aunt who is substituting for the grandmother says that when Elisa hears the grandmother's name spoken she begins looking for her* (seven and a half months).

The grandmother thinks that Elisa needs a lot of affection. During the sextuplets' first year she rocks her to sleep almost every evening (nine and a half months). This little girl prefers to go to sleep alone without the other sextuplets, so she stays in the grandparents' room and is put in the bedroom with the others only after she is asleep (12½ months).

Elisa never sucks her thumb and does not want a dummy (eight and a half months).

At 15 months she weighs only six and a half kilos.

She is the last of the sextuplets to get her first tooth, at 11 months, and she begins to walk at about 15 months.

## Sociability

Elisa is a vivacious, friendly and affectionate little girl who frequently and actively seeks contact with adults, including the observer.

*Elisa is sitting on the lap of an aunt who is talking to her, and she responds, making noises and kicking and moving her arms energetically* (seven and a half months).

Elisa and Franco are always the first to notice the arrival of visitors. They attract attention with their big smiles and agitated movements, and the adults make friendly comments. *As soon as the observer comes into the room, Franco turns around in the play-pen, stands up and jumps up and down joyfully. Elisa, in a child seat, watches the scene, and soon she, too, moves her arms and legs, squealing* (nine and a half months).

*Elisa is standing alone in a play-pen watching the other sextuplets. She looks at the observer with cheerful eyes and raises her right hand as if to greet her* (13½ months).

She is inventive and knows how to amuse herself. *Elisa makes the mother understand that she wants to stand in the net shopping bag attached to the handles of the stroller. "That's her favourite position," the mother says. As soon as she is put there Elisa begins to chatter vivaciously, looking all around satisfied* (14 months).

*Elisa notices the observer's arrival; she smiles and jumps towards the gate exclaiming, "Oo-oo"* (19 months).

*When the observer arrives, Elisa immediately goes towards her offering her a piece of a construction toy. The observer says hello, Elisa begins to make gurgling sounds, and then offers another piece of the toy* (21 months).

*The observer enters the living room where the mother is sitting on a cushion on the floor; Alice is next to her with a small telephone in her hand. Elisa immediately goes towards the observer and gives her a ball saying, "Ball, ball, ball." Then she points to an armchair and says, "Grandpa, Ggrandpa." The mother explains that that is where the grandfather always sits. Then Elisa goes toward another armchair and says, "Daddy, Daddy". The mother comments, "Mummy and Grandma don't have chairs because they are always on their feet"* (22 months).

She even asks the observer for help. *Franco pulls off the hat that Elisa is wearing and throws it down triumphantly, then gallops off towards the living room. Elisa seems sad and offended; she picks up the hat, takes it to the observer, puts it in her hand and lowers her head so that she can put it back on for her* (23 months).

*The grandmother recounts that the children saw themselves on television in a programme about them that lasted 20 minutes. After recognizing herself, Elisa called out, "Eli, Eli"* (two years and two months).

*The grandmother alerts the children when the observer arrives. "Look who's here. It's our lady friend." Elisa runs to the observer, stops just in front of her and smiles affectionately* (two years and four months).

It is easy for Elisa to find company because of her spontaneous attachment to adults, her vivacity and her interest in life. She is so sociable and able to establish new relationships that she becomes the favourite of a 15-year-old neighbour, "Elisa's friend", who often comes to the house to play with her.

*When her "friend" comes in, Elisa gets excited and reaches out her arms. The girl picks up a small pink jacket and a hat with lace trimming and puts them on Elisa, who looks like a doll. "She's small, but she's all there!" exclaims the grandmother, and the adolescent and little girl couple go out for a walk* (16 months).

## Conflicts and contrasts

Sometimes there are violent clashes between Elisa and the mother. The mother claims that the little girl looks like her own younger brother.

*Elisa gets her 15-year-old "friend" to take her out of the house; they go to the piazza and then head towards the church. "Pray, pray," says the mother sarcastically* (18 months).

The observation begins with the sound of Elisa's crying and the mother yelling: "Stupid." *The sextuplets are returning home from a walk. Alice sits down on the ground and the mother says hastily: "Let's go or I'll leave you here in the street!" The little girl fusses; the mother asks the observer to push her in the push-chair while she goes to get the other "stubborn" one, Elisa, who is then put in the push-chair next to Alice. As soon as they arrive home, Elisa begins to cry and tries to get out of the push-chair. The mother lets Alice get out and asks the observer to help Elisa, who doesn't want to stand up and kicks and cries furiously. The mother leaves her lying on the concrete and yells: "If you don't stop, you'll drive us crazy! Ugly, little skinny thing!"* (20 months).

*The mother notices all of a sudden that Elisa has her pen and she immediately confronts her yelling: "You wretch! Who gave you that? You mustn't take my things!" She grabs it away from her and goes to put it back in her own room* (two years and three months).

Elisa sometimes teases her brothers. *Daniele, with a dummy in his mouth, pulls himself up on his feet and leans on the child seat where Elisa is sitting. She immediately takes the dummy from his mouth, and plays with it putting it in her own mouth. Daniele stands there with his tongue out, touching first his lips with his hands and then the edge of the child seat. Elisa waves the dummy in his face and, almost by chance, he manages to grab it and put it back in his mouth. Elisa takes it away again and Daniele, looking surprised, is left with his tongue dangling out of his mouth* (nine and a half months).

## Brunet-Lezine test (14 months, 18 days)

Elisa and Bruno do the tests in the afternoon while the others are out. Elisa is first because Bruno suddenly refuses to take the test. She takes her mother's hand and walks into the room with her.

After the examiner puts out the blocks, Elisa picks up one and holds it tightly in her hand while playing with the other two. Then she puts all three on the table and begins a sort of conversation; she is particularly interested in one block and uses it to push the other two around. (Here we detect a symbolic game that can be linked to the concept of sibling Oedipal triangles which we discuss further on in chapter IV, paragraph 4). When the examiner shows her a tower, she immediately makes one herself with two blocks. She fills the cup with blocks. She uses the spoon pretending to eat and to feed the mother. Then she has fun making a noise by moving the spoon around in the cup. She is quick at taking the tablet out of the bottle, putting it back in and taking it out again.

The examiner writes: "All her movements are intentional; nothing happens by chance. She responds as foreseen by the test." She immediately makes the bell ring and pulls the napkin away "deliberately". She plays with the table board and the round piece, but copies the examiner immediately once she has demonstrated how to insert the latter into the board. She also imitates by scribbling with the pencil.

At the end of the test the grandmother asks: "How did my pet do?"

## At the nursery school (two years, nine months, 12 days)

Elisa continues to be sociable and extroverted. She notices immediately the arrival of the observer, and smiles at her both then and when she leaves. Elisa plays animatedly and is friendly with an older girl whose hand she holds happily. Unlike her sister, Elisa accepts the role of the little girl when the older one asks her to do so, and she accepts pretending to be fed like a baby.

## Personality traits and relational characteristics

In the first observation Elisa is presented to the observer by the grandmother. The mother thinks Elisa resembles her own younger brother, suggesting a maternal projection of childhood conflicts connected with feelings of jealousy and sibling rivalry.

During early infancy Elisa is left mostly to the care of the grandmother with whom she establishes a strong bond. She appears capable of finding alternative solutions rather than competing, for example with her sister. She shows a remarkable capacity for socializing with others even outside the family environment, and actively seeks relationships with non-family adults. Although for the mother she is the less favoured of the two daughters, Elisa seems to adapt to this reality, reacting positively and developing her own personal capabilities. She presents the typical behaviour of the youngest child (see Sulloway, 1997) who, through adaptability, originality, and ingenuity cultivates different abilities to reduce competition with the "firstborn" sister to a minimum.

## Franco: The baby boy

Franco was the last of the sextuplets to be born, with a birth weight of 1550 grams. When he was taken home for the first time, he weighed 2980 grams. After a short time in the hospital because at home he cried continually, he returned home weighing 3390 grams. He was the only sextuplet to have such an experience.

He underwent surgery for inguinal hernia like his brothers Carlo and Daniele.

Neuromotor-relational evaluation (one and a half months): "It is impossible to evaluate psycho-motor function at this time because he is still under the influence of the anaesthesia and the shock of the surgery."

### First impressions

Franco is the first of the sextuplets the observer meets because he is the only child who is awake and in the kitchen with the mother and the grandmother as they chat and go about their cooking chores (*"il beato tra le donne"*, an Italian expression referring to a man pleasantly surrounded by women).

*Franco is in the child seat on the kitchen table. As the observer enters he takes a good look at her. Every once in a while the mother calls him and he responds with smiles and gurgles kicking his feet* (six and a half months).

He responds readily to external stimuli.

*He and all the other sextuplets are in their prams ready to visit a neighbour who has a big garden. He stretches his legs, pushing them against the side of the pram, then stares at the light coming through the trees and kicks his feet making happy noises and little shrieks* (seven and a half months).

*The observer enters the living room with one of the children's aunts. Franco, who is sitting in a play-pen, turns around immediately, then stands up. When the aunt introduces him to the observer he gets excited and flexes his knees back and forth* (eight and a half months).

*Elisa and Franco are the first to notice the arrival of visitors who are immediately attracted to them. The two children first smile then laugh and dance about as the adults make some friendly conversation with both of them* (nine and a half months).

## Relationship with the mother

The mother is not worried about this sextuplet: she controls him less than the other babies and behaves in a more relaxed manner with him as if she has more trust in him than in the others. She treats him as if he were a child who knows how to take care of himself and she takes pride in him. This mother-baby relationship seems to be based on a solid alliance, perhaps even on some unspoken secret agreement.

*Happy to get out of the push-chairs, the children run into the fenced garden. The mother goes to Franco and shows him a ramp that he can use to run up and down. Franco runs towards the ramp enthusiastically* (18 months).

*The helper alerts the mother that lunch will be ready in a few minutes. The mother whispers in Franco's ear: "Go to Grandma for your lunch"* (22 months).

*Franco is about to hit Bruno. "No, give your brother a nice pat," says the mother who is sitting with the children on the living room floor. Franco repeats "Nice pat" and transforms his gesture into a caress [...]. The mother takes Franco to be changed; he looks happy to be washed. As she rubs the cream on his genitals he stares at Mummy and laughs with all his heart. She then puts her face close to his and asks, "Where's your little thing?" Then she takes his penis between her fingers and pretends to show it to him. He is attentive and enthralled. Then the mother dresses him quickly and says, "Now you're ready for lunch." As soon as he is back on his feet on the floor Franco jumps up and down energetically with both legs together* (23 months).

However, there can also be violent clashes with the mother. *The mother and the children are out for a walk with the helper. Daniele runs ahead, and when he reaches a pile of gravel along the road he sits down and digs his hands into it. Franco notices his brother's discovery and runs off to do the same. The mother calls them and they stop what they are doing, look up but don't take their hands out of the gravel. The mother picks Franco up, carries him away and sits him down with her on a doorstep. Carlo passes*

*near them. All of a sudden the mother gives Franco two slaps and a severe*
*scolding. Franco cries so hard he turns blue. The mother says he is "stupid*
*and dumb": at this point Franco seems desperate and disconsolate and looks*
*at his mother, shaking and sweating profusely. The mother says that Franco*
*is fussy and has too many tantrums. After a while when both Franco and*
*the mother have calmed down, the mother's mood changes and she hugs*
*him affectionately* (two years and a half months).

## Sociability

Franco, like Elisa, notices right away when the observer arrives and
he often stops what he is doing to give some sign of recognition,
such as a smile or a friendly gesture.

*When Franco sees the observer he gives her big smiles and then turns his*
*head around repeatedly as if he wants to play peek-a-boo* (12½ months).

*Alice is sucking on a carrot and stares at the observer without greet-*
*ing her, but Franco immediately raises his head and smiles cunningly*
(16 months).

*As soon as the observer arrives, Franco raises his head, smiles, and shows*
*her two rubber blocks that he hits together energetically* (19 months).

*Franco rides the tricycle around the observer and then rides off towards*
*the hall* (two years and six months).

Similar to Elisa who has been chosen as the favourite child by
an adolescent girl, Franco is the favourite of a neighbour who often
comes to help at meal times and wants to feed him.

*A neighbour comes in and offers to help out before she goes to do her*
*shopping. The grandmother says they don't need any help for now, but the*
*woman picks up Franco and doesn't appear willing to leave before he has been*
*fed. She waits while the mother takes him to be changed, but Franco fusses*
*because, according to the mother, he doesn't want to stay on the changing*
*table. Then, while she buttons up his trousers, she asks him where Daddy is*
*and Franco points at the picture on the wall. She then asks where Mummy*
*is and Franco again points at the picture of the father, and the mother jokes*
*that he doesn't know the difference between them. The neighbour who is*
*waiting patiently now picks up "the baby boy"* (the observer's perception, see table 1) *and takes him into the kitchen* (15 months).

*At lunch time the neighbour arrives to help out. The grandmother tells*
*her to finish feeding Daniele and the woman sits down in the grandmother's*
*chair. Franco immediately goes and stands at her feet, while she is feeding*

*his brother. A few minutes later Franco begins to cry and the neighbour tries unsuccessfully to console him. Franco goes into a rage, crying angrily and pulling at the woman's clothes* (16 months).

*Franco's eyes light up when the neighbour enters. He pretends to hide and she does the same. The mother says, "Franco, look who's here!" He runs up to the woman and she takes him in her arms. She complains about the cold weather that is bothering her, and then the two women talk about the death of a common acquaintance* (24 months).

Again, like Elisa, for a while Franco sleeps in the grandparents' room.

*It has become a habit for Franco to go to sleep on a travel cot in the grandparents' room* (8th, 11th, 12th and 13th observations).

## Play

Franco is original, inventive, and assertive in play; he freely expresses his emotions and feelings, ranging widely from affectionate to aggressive and in certain moments appears to be pensive.

*The grandmother tells the observer that Franco and Daniele like to be together. "Daniele sucks on a dummy a lot and Franco often grabs it out of his mouth"* (11 months).

*Franco is intent on playing a game with the observer that he has invented and directs: he places some plastic toys in her hands and then quickly takes them back. Suddenly he notices that the other sextuplets have biscuits and he runs off to the kitchen with his hands on his hips (a sign of indignation). The grandmother comments: "He's the cleverest"* (15 months).

*During the morning walk Franco is paired with Daniele to whom he pays no attention, apparently preferring to invent his own game: as he sings to himself he alternates clapping his hands with slapping them on his knees* (18 months).

*When she arrives the observer finds the children all in the big garden next door. Franco and Elisa notice her right away and they both smile and start jumping towards the gate exclaiming, "Oo-oo". Franco shows the observer two rubber blocks that he hits together energetically [...]. Daniele, a dummy in his mouth, runs back and forth with a red bucket in his hand. Franco walks to the centre of the garden, sits down and builds a tower with the rubber blocks. His brother runs over to him, knocks down the tower, and carries away one of the blocks. Franco, surprised and stunned, becomes angry and cries desperately. He gets up and goes towards the house. The grandmother goes to him, picks him up and tries to console him.*

*(After, in the house) Franco finds the box of nappies under the table and invents a game: he takes the nappies one at a time to the door with the missing glass and throws them on the other side of the door. The grandmother tells him to stop; he listens to her, looks at the nappy in his hand, and then decides to continue and throws it* (19 months).

*Franco is busy putting his foot in a box. Carlo tries to imitate him, but his foot gets stuck and he begins to cry. Franco looks at him for a moment, then continues playing. [...] The father comes in and the children all run to greet him. Then they go back to their play. Franco returns to where he was in the middle of the living room and looks attentively at the pictures in a book, as if he were studying them. Daniele, imitating him, finds a piece of paper with figures on it and looks at it. Carlo passes by and grabs the paper out of his hand, and Daniele lets out a scream* (21 months).

*Franco notices the light indicating that the washing machine is on and he has fun covering it with his hand and then taking his hand away. Alice comes over and with the air of an adult points at the light and says to her brother, "Boo-boo." Franco pays no attention to her and continues to play* (23 months).

*Bruno is playing with a wooden box, putting different shaped pieces into it. All of a sudden Franco stops moving around in the little toy car, directs himself towards his brother and tries to grab the toy away from him. Bruno protests and says, distinguishing the sounds, "Sca-to-la"* (the Italian word for box). *Franco insists, but Bruno manages to keep hold of the box. The mother quickly gets another box and offers it to Franco so that he will leave the other one for Bruno. Franco accepts happily* (24 months).

*Daniele tries to grab a tube away from Franco. Franco becomes angry, stamps his feet on the floor and agitates his arms, practically scaring his brother who lets the tube fall to the floor as he runs away. [...] When Bruno puts on a record, Franco twirls around and around by himself so fast that he gets dizzy and then, rather amused, lets himself fall on the ground [...]. The helper announces: "Here's some water. Who wants a drink?" The sextuplets all go to her, get in a line and start to drink, one at a time. All of a sudden Franco pushes ahead of the others in order to get his drink faster* (25 months).

*Franco notices that the father has given his hand to Carlo and he wants it also, but the father says no; Franco throws himself down on the floor, lays still for a few minutes and then goes back to his playing* (two years and three months).

*Carlo tries to close the curtains of the living room window and the mother scolds him: "Go away, don't make it dark." Franco goes up to his brother, gives him a strong push and Carlo starts crying but doesn't open the curtains"* (two years and four months).

### Brunet-Lezine test (14 months, 18 days)

The mother decides that he should be the first one to do the test, saying that she is sure he "will be able to do it". In fact, Franco begins spontaneously to build a tower with the two blocks, meanwhile making "various noises in a voice full of inflexion and expression". It is recorded that he "looks at the examiner and the mother, who smiles and encourages him". He continues doing the trials satisfactorily, showing initiative and willingness to follow the examiner's indications. At a certain point he tries to take the examiner's pen and the mother comments with satisfaction: "He's a show-off and pays attention to the reactions of adults."

In the last trial he seems to want to direct things: he "takes the pencil, puts it in his mouth and then hits it down on the sheet of paper". The examiner tries to take the pencil to show him how to write, but he will not give it up, forcing her to get another one to scribble with. Franco takes the examiner's pencil and makes dots on the paper.

At the end of the test he leaves the room on tiptoe.

### At the nursery school (two years, nine months, 12 days)

Franco is interested in playing and shows a lot of initiative. He asks for adult help when he needs it; for example, to go to the lavatory. He invents a game with the pistol, attracting the attention of the other sextuplets, and he becomes the leader of the group. He accepts the frustrating interference of the teacher and knows how to wait his turn to get the pistol back and continue his play in which he freely expresses anger and aggressiveness.

### Personality traits and relational characteristics

Franco is the baby boy whose company the mother seems to enjoy; she is not particularly worried about him and behaves in a more relaxed and less demanding way. Franco is vivacious, sociable, and interested in people and the world around him. He plays joyfully, is full of inventiveness, and is ready to include his siblings. These relational characteristics seem to be indicative of synchrony between a mother who is available and relaxed (less of a school teacher) and a child who is sufficiently independent and competent. Brazelton (1990, p. 122) says that good child-parent synchronous communication helps the child to feel he has a reliable, willing parent and the parent to feel competent and sure of him- or herself. This seems to have been favoured by the parents' acceptance of the boy's identification with certain of the father's characteristics: like being affectionate and patient, not demanding, and sensitive to the difficulties others have. This undoubtedly contributed to the possibility of negotiating the Oedipal conflict and integrating aggression towards and rivalry with the other sextuplet siblings.

Franco seems to have developed his own personalized capacity for positive self-affirmation and is well adapted to the family environment.

*CHAPTER FOUR*

# Being in six

H aving given the history of the first three years of life of the sextuplets and the personality profiles of each child, all based on the observations, we now proceed with a more in-depth investigation into certain significant aspects of relationships within the family.

## *An atypical maternal identity*

For every new mother, acquiring a new identity involves ambivalent feelings, at times hostile and painful, that she must learn to tolerate, cope with and, eventually, integrate into her own personal identity. One notes in this young woman's pre-motherhood history various conflictual experiences involving complex issues such as sexuality and becoming an adult, as well as her acceptance of this unusual pregnancy (see chapter II, paragraphs 1 and 2). She recounts that she did not consider herself normal because of her "misfortune" in being sterile, and that she had thought that she was being "deprived" of motherhood. During the hormone treatments she became more hyperactive than usual: she took long, solitary walks or bicycle rides and she took up painting, writing poetry, and

73

knitting. She remembers that when she was younger she did not want children. She was afraid because her pregnancy and mother-hood were linked, and almost equated in her mind, to the obesity against which she had fought so hard during adolescence until she became anorexic which possibly influenced her capacity to be fer-tile. Her anorexia was probably a way of managing the psychologi-cal weight of her maturative issues, leading to infertility, the need to control things, and the lack of desire to have babies inside her. She claims to have been glad every time the fertility treatment failed. Though attributing her pregnancy to a well-conducted scientific procedure, she also felt that it had deprived her of the emotions normally experienced by other women.

This atypical pregnancy and motherhood, to some extent imposed on her and in any case traumatic, became a dramatic challenge for survival, not only in relation to external reality. The number of foetuses may have increased this woman's anxieties, fears and ambivalence about motherhood. On a fantasy level, the birth of twins, triplets etc. may incite, in the mother especially, "the anguish of being a prey for nature" (Lecourt, 2003, p. 176) and may be associated with feelings of animalism and even monstrosity. We mentioned (chapter II, paragraph 2, "Pregnancy and delivery") that the c. 30 kilos weight increase aroused persecutory fantasies, as the mother herself recounted.

After the birth of the sextuplets the mother, to maintain group cohesion, becomes the manager of the family organization as well as the absolute, indisputable chief director. Her professional identity as a competent teacher helps her maintain an overall view of the children's developmental processes and their educational needs. The desire to differentiate between the sextuplets and to individuate their different characteristics and capabilities is related not only to the need to maintain control over the group, but also to have a per-sonalized relationship with each one. As we shall see further on, the children seem to adapt to the mother's need to differentiate between them, insofar as is possible for individuals who are and feel part of such a special group.

Both psychically and physically the mother experienced her preg-nancy and motherhood as a tumultuous and somewhat hostile real-ity that besieged her both internally and externally, arousing such strong feelings of vulnerability that she felt that her very integrity was threatened (chapter II, paragraph 2, "Pregnancy and delivery"). To avoid feeling this internal reality, the mother seems to experience a "flight toward a fantasy of omnipotence" (Winnicott, 1935), finding reassurance in the role of super-mother, becoming a sort of "movie star" with a large audience kept up-to-date by the media. At other times stress, tiredness, and desperation took hold and she was prey to negative, self-denigrating, persecutory thoughts: for example, when the mother arrives regularly after the observer, when she criticizes the observer for not doing anything ("here we need more hands than eyes" fourth observation), and when she complains because she feels misunderstood by people who invent stories about her and accuse her unjustly of taking advantage of welfare assistance.

One can well understand the mother's manic self-defence given her early history of anorexia, fear of sexuality and motherhood and the inherent difficulties of her very burdensome and exceptional situation. This threatening and dangerous "flight from internal reality" (Winnicott, 1935) is based on the primitive mechanism of denial (Klein, 1932) that seems to have helped her accept the sextuplet group as a reality. We note, for example, her reaction when she is told she is carrying six babies: "All or none!" Then again how else could she have mentally grasped the meaning of such an incomparable and non-human situation? The help and support of the maternal grandmother seems to have permitted the mother to turn to her professional identity in relating to the children and that, too, contributed to the stability and continuity of the relationships within the family group as a whole. This made it possible for her to find a way to establish satisfactory, gratifying relationships with the children.

There was another period of crisis at the beginning of the second winter when "the children were everywhere" (see chapter II, paragraph 11); the mother could not return to her teaching job and was forced to stay at home to care for them. At this point her omnipotent defences crumbled and there were clear signs of a delayed postpartum depression.

## Being part of a homogeneous group

The sextuplet's experience of being part of a group, which began before birth, was to be of structural value in their psychic development as individuals.

During their life in the uterus, the sextuplets shared a common world and lived prematurely in a group environment. As with an animal litter where the puppies or cubs help each other, finding stimulation and wellbeing through physical contact and shared body heat, the sextuplets underwent a process of "natural" adaptation, in which staying with others precedes the need for attachment to a mothering figure. "Being brothers or sisters implies the tranquillizing warmth of a strong, sweet bond of satisfying relationship with others like oneself so similar that they cannot be distinguished one from another" (Brunori, 1996, p. 118). The prenatal experience of sharing tactile-auditory sensations (Maiello, 1993) becomes a primary source of communication that fosters strong group cohesion among such children.

Piontelli's (1992) longitudinal observational and psychoanalytical studies show surprising coherence in the psychology and behaviour of the individual as a foetus, baby and child. In particular, in the case of pregnancies with more than one foetus, using ultrasound she observed that the foetuses relate to one another and described how certain twins are actively hostile to one another while others have more harmonious relationships, and that the characteristics of such relationships continue after birth.

Just as the birth signified separation from the mother's body, simultaneously the precocious interaction between the sextuplets was interrupted. Immediately after their birth, although they were not subjected to intensive hospital care, the six babies were separated from one another and thus experienced a form of isolation.

Once they were all home the prenatal state of being an exclusive group of six turned into actually living together with others in a family environment and interacting daily with a mother, a father, grandparents and various helpers as well as among themselves.

The question is whether or not being part of a twin-triplet … sextuplet sibling group can compensate for a child's need to have the mother all for him/herself. A newborn needs the individual attention of a carer (see the studies on the effects of institutionalization of infants). Were our sextuplets lonely babies deprived of the maternal breast?

Our investigation of the affective-relational life of the sextuplets included research and review of studies about the influence of sibling relationships on individual psychic structure and development.

As early as 1927, Buhler described overlapping situations of symmetry and projection among three-year-olds, observing that children show empathy in attributing their own emotions to other children of the same age (for example, a child cries when he sees another child fall). She further emphasized the dependence of children less than a year old on images of their peers. Buhler obtained her information from observations during her paediatric out-patient practice. She observed babies of the same age together while they sat in the waiting room with their mothers, noting that their motor reactions were directly influenced by those of their peers.

These pioneer studies, together with the practically simultaneous ones done by Wallon in France who studied the inter-relationship between biological and social factors in psychic development and the perception of the self in early infancy (*"stade du miroir"* or mirror stage), were the starting point for evolutional psychology and infant researches. These have amply documented the existence of early communication and imitation between babies that represent the very beginning of social understanding (Dunn, 1985). Then in the second year, babies go from affective resonance (Stern, 1985), when they are upset by others, to behaviour that demonstrates their interest in the suffering of a sibling and the capacity to put themselves in the place of the other and to try to comfort him. In the third year they react to explicit manifestations of another child's emotions, such as states of sadness or anger. Also in the sphere of sibling conflict, children often show clearly their capability to bother or provoke another individual.

These studies demonstrate that the central element of emotional and social development in children in the first three years is not limited to relationships with the mother or the parents. Instead, we note that the continuous presence of a child different from oneself, one who is even too well-known and who is in competition for the affection and attention of the parents, may be very important for the development of a child's sense of self, his feelings of security and his capacity to understand others (Dunn and Plomin, 1990). To build self-esteem, the child needs the loving attention of the mother as well as that of his siblings (Cooper and Magagna, 2005).

Also in the fields of psychodynamics and psychoanalysis, where research on this topic is still limited (for a general review of sibling relationships see Brunori, 1997; Algini, 2003; Mori, 2004), identification with a sibling is recognized to have a fundamental role in psychic development. In addition to the mother-child couple, also others (the father, older siblings, grandparents, etc.) play an important role in promoting the differentiation between self and non-self. Neubauer (1982) refers to early multiple interactions that can determine different evolutional phases leading to the integration of ego functions, and affirms that the problem is not only one of rivalry with a third object (father or sibling), but that the child tends to incorporate and imitate the mother's behaviour towards others, whether through altruistic surrender or competition. Leichtman (1985) observed strong mutual attachment between siblings before the sixth month of life; he believes that sometimes children understand each other better than the parents understand them. In a longitudinal study done by the Yale University Study Group on the development of pre-school age siblings and how they influence each other, Kris and Ritvo (1983) emphasize that a child who has negotiated sibling rivalry is more advanced in coping with frustration and Oedipal rivalry.

In their study on large families, Bossard and Bell (1956) affirmed that when parents are tired and burdened with responsibility without sufficient energy or affective resources to satisfy their children's emotional needs, the children often seek out their siblings. Even in so-called extreme situations of deficient parental care there may develop a compensatory pattern that tends to reinforce the bond between siblings (Bank, 1982), which may lead to bonds of friendship among them such that the sibling group becomes the main source of affection. Such a compensatory pattern consolidates a strong group identity in which the development of the self takes place through wider spread rather than deep relationships.

A community of children produces horizontal relationships that may predispose towards the recognition of a need for dependence and reciprocity. Thus it becomes possible to consider the other as a peer and to develop a capacity for identification (Freud, 1921). M. Klein (1932) talked about secret complicity between siblings against adults, "we" opposed to "they", which helps the child to distance himself from the parent, promoting emotional development.

This strong sibling bond can have a determining role in any love relationship even later in adult life. M. Harris (1987) affirms that among different age siblings certain brothers or sisters may attract more admiration and dependence, and even imitation, than the parents. The friendship between siblings, based on the experience of growing up together, can produce an intimate understanding and affection with a peer of the opposite sex that helps one make a wise choice of a spouse (which is our personal wish for these sextuplets). P. Coles (2003) reminds us of sibling influence on personality development, a topic that has been neglected and poorly explored in clinical psychoanalysis, and the importance of the sibling in one's internal world, emphasizing the necessity to consider the phenomenon of sibling transference in clinical situations.

In the discussion following the seventh observation (12½ months) it was pointed out that the sextuplets were not aggressive children, that they showed limited antagonistic reactions towards one another, giving the impression that they lived in a cushioned environment of appeasement. Bettelheim (1969) noticed that children living in a *kibbutz* showed limited aggressiveness and strong dependence on their peer group. He wondered if the limited aggressiveness evidenced might not depend on the fact that the children spent little time with their parents. The sextuplets did not eat voraciously and asked little of the adults. They did not fight much with each other and their tantrums were few and brief.

Although well cared for, the sextuplets are inevitably conditioned by the circumstances: there is less individual time with the mother and more time with other carers and with each other, less time for intimacy and few possibilities for being alone. Each sextuplet has to learn to accept an intermittent mother-child relationship. Maintaining a relationship with a mother who is always busy and must be shared with so many others requires remarkable capacities for tolerating frustration and adapting to reality. The impossibility of having exclusive relationships with the mother forced the sextuplets to learn self-limitation which, in turn, helped to avoid the risk of ruining group cohesion. When a child accepts the quantity of maternal love available, the experience of sibling relationships can be a good basis for narcissism wherein self-esteem and object love can co-exist without excessive conflict.

Studies on sibling relationships show that evenly distributed maternal attention diminishes rivalry and aggression, and actually favours affectionate behaviour among siblings. Furthermore, mothers who are not antagonistic in their behaviour with their children and who do not get overly involved in their children's sibling hostilities, create an atmosphere that favours pro-social behaviour in the children. Using E. Bick's *Infant Observation* methodology in her research on sibling bonds, D. Vallino (2004) observed that the mother's (and father's) capacity to relate to their children by recognizing individual qualities can transform feelings of jealousy and rivalry among siblings and promote a process of identification between them. Thus, the sibling experience becomes one of emotional learning about others, which exerts positive influences on development, enriching the individual while excessive parental involvement in sibling relationships can have a disturbing influence and weaken sibling loyalty (Bank and Kahn, 1982). Even the attachment theory supports the idea that there is a tie between good parental care and good sibling relationships.

Studying attachment relationships in rhesus monkeys, Suomi (1982) observed that under experimental conditions baby monkeys separated from their biological mothers are anxious and withdrawn, but if they are put into the care of a substitute "supermother" and brought up with other "siblings" rather than alone, which is their natural condition, their behavioural repertoire grows more rapidly in the sense that they have positive reactions and are more sociable with the other monkeys from whom they receive support. Suomi believes that humans can have reactions similar to those of non-human primates. This corresponds with what we observed in the development of our group of sextuplets in that each child's evolutional course was influenced by growing up together from the time of conception.

Although, on one hand, being part of a sextuplet group has a "cushion effect" on the personality development of the six children, on the other it may foster altruistic behaviour among them (Dunn and Boer, 1992). Subsequently the sibling group may have a supportive role in the Oedipal drama, as is widely recognized in studies on this subject.

These sextuplets have a capacity for sharing and socializing among themselves. They show a particularly affectionate attachment to each other; what P. Coles (2003) calls "brotherly love": a non-incestuous love that gives each one support while shaping ways to relate to others in adult life. Over the years the bond between the sextuplets seem to have become a fundamental element in their individual personalities and favoured dependence on the group with a function similar to that observed in adolescent peer groups (Meltzer, 1979).

As Bion (1961) says, personal identity implies structurally a group dimension: the survival of the group depends on the need of each member to remain a part of it, and belonging to a group can be a pleasant experience as well as a defence against psychotic anxieties of disintegration and fragmentation.

## The mother-child-sextuplet group relationship

Research on triplets-quadruplets-quintuplets-sextuplets evidence that in such cases the mothers have attachment difficulties and tend to be less involved with their children (Garrel, 1992, 1994, 1997), not only because of lack of time, fatigue, and psychological stress, but because they experience greater ambivalence towards offspring of births involving more than two babies (Goshen-Gottstein, 1980). The interactions between the mothers and such groups of children involve mostly the numerous tasks that must be carried out. Notwithstanding the need to give equal care to all the children and keep them all calm and under control, the mothers of such sibling groups have difficulty in building a relationship with more than one child; they need to differentiate the children, one from another, to be able to relate to each one as a distinct individual (Robins and Anderson, 1991).

It is well known that unconscious parental attitudes and attributions (*Unconscious Labels*, Brazelton and Cramer, 1990) exist regarding children's characteristics, and that these unconscious labels influence caretaking. A method of attribution of personal characteristics, so called de-twinning or de-tripleting … etc. (Zazzo, 1984), allows parents of twins-triplets … sextuplets to behave differently with each child and allows the children to respond accordingly. Studies on the strategies used by parents of multiple births show that the strategy of attachment to the children as a group includes differentiation between the children through labeling based on their individual personalities (Robins and Anderson, 1991).

The mothers can become attached to the group as a unit rather than to the individual children, or form a preferential bond with one child to the detriment of the others. They can be very afraid of the consequences of favouritism or exclusive attachment to only one of the many children because preferential treatment can cause hostility among the children. We noted above, for example, how in the 13th observation the mother recognizes the danger of having sent Alice to the seaside with the grandparents, "She got used to being alone, and we can't allow that."

The relational model established in this family from the very beginning was that of a group of adults who took care of a group of children within a matriarchal family structure, an organization imposed by the dramatic situation.

We have prepared four diagrams that give a graphic representation of the mother-child-sextuplet group relationships to help the reader visualize this unique situation.

As long as the children were small and could be treated more or less in the same way inasmuch as their needs were basically the same, that is as a sort of homogeneous nestling-group with minimal individual problems, the mother managed the situation well enough with rapid group-directed activities based on a sort of globalized overview. We note her later regret when she mentions in her book that, back in those early months, meal times meant feeding the children in an assembly line fashion using a single dish and only one spoon (Figure 1).

This phase lasted until the children were about a year old, when illnesses, sleeping problems, and alimentary idiosyncrasies began

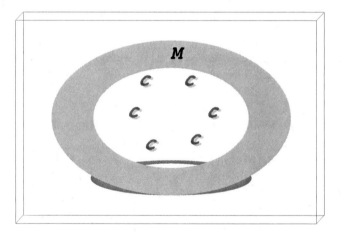

Figure 1. Unity: The mother managed the children as a group.

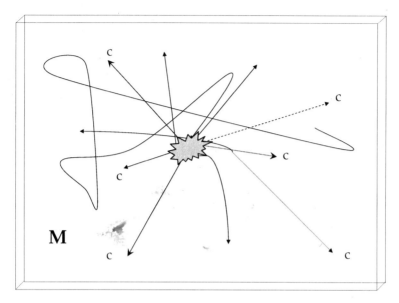

Figure 2.  Chaos: The children were everywhere.

to set in and disturb the daily routine. At about the same time the sextuplets started to walk, making it even more difficult to manage them as a group. The mother now had to cope with the unacceptable reality of individual needs and requests. Afraid that they would cause trouble or that a sort of "diaspora" would occur, she tried with all her might to keep them together as much as possible and constantly under control, but, alas, "They were everywhere" (Figure 2).

This family situation, similar to that of a community under the continual threat of chaos and the risk of explosion due to the overwhelming number of simultaneous demands, meant that the children had to learn self-control, adapt to being part of a group-world and accept start-and-stop relationships with the mother. Each child had to learn to share the mother with the other five siblings. No one could be treated as a single child at the centre of the mother's attention for more than a few minutes at a time. This meant having only one-sixth of a mother and limiting each's needs and requests, as may easily happen with six siblings of different ages (Figure 3).

The mother could not allow herself to show preferences for any of the children, and they in turn were not allowed to rebel. Different

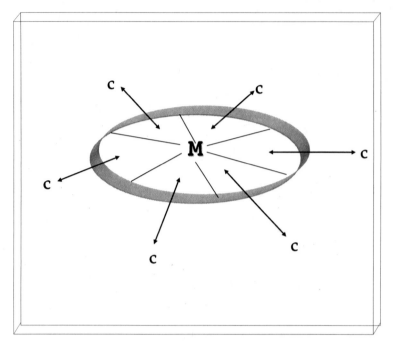

Figure 3. Sharing: Each child had one-sixth of the mother.

from the situation with twins or triplets, where the children manage to have more of the same mother, the sextuplets seemed to have various other mother figures at different times: the mother, the grandmother, the helpers, the neighbour women, and the other relatives. There were no reports of and we did not observe the sextuplets refusing any of the mother substitutes. Adaptation, thus, implicated accepting primary care from whoever was available and renouncing exclusive care from the mother (Figure 4).

However, although they shared the same intra-uterine space, from birth the sextuplets have occupied a very different space in the mother's mind and each one has had a unique relationship with her. The relationships with the other adult carer figures are not interchangeable with those, necessarily intermittent and short-lived, with the mother.

The way the mother coped with certain tasks common to all mothers highlights how making the most simple decision can become a problem with so many children all the same age. For example, she

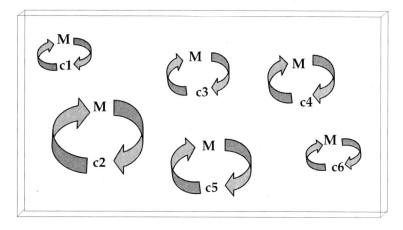

Figure 4. Exclusive relationships: Each child had limited and brief one-to-one contact with the mother.

found a very original solution to her wish to make photo albums for the children to document their childhood. Realizing that it would be impossible for her to make six separate albums, one for each child, she decided to make a single family album for each year, numbering them progressively. In this way each child would have a volume of photographs related to a specific period. Thus the mother, quite aware of the difficulties imposed on her by the sextuplets, found a most original solution that was fair to all concerned while reinforcing the unity of the sextuplet group.

## Diversity: The search for a niche

We have seen how the mother reacted differently to each sextuplet and that she perceived each one as a distinct individual. This allowed each child to have its own personal experiences, different from those of the other sextuplets.

In their studies on the differences between siblings and the factors that influence their relationships, Dunn and Plomin (1990) suggest that non-shared situations have the greatest influence on personality. According to their theory, environmental influences are different for each child within the same family, both regarding how the parents treat the children as well as how the children react to differentiated treatment depending on their temperaments and personalities. Therefore, the environmental factors most important for development are those that children experience differently within the same family, as regards parental influence, age, and sex differences of siblings, birth order, individual roles within the family, family dynamics, and life events. Alfred Adler (1928) was one of the first to study the importance of birth order. The studies for his theories on the psychology of the individual included research on the influence of birth order and the position and role of siblings within the family group on the development of personality. Although our group of sextuplets were brought up in the same family, each of the children had its own subjective experiences not shared by the others. And this repeated experience of specific and differing relationships with their various carers contributed to establishing behavioural patterns and relational styles which became internalized during the course of development.

According to the personality theory proposed by evolutional psychology, which emphasizes the importance of biology, the differences between siblings exemplifies the Darwinian principle of divergence that allows the species to compete for limited resources. Diversification between siblings encourages the development of different capabilities and interests, contributing to reduce direct competition making coexistence and, consequently, survival possible. The search for a niche within the family is a useful strategy among siblings that reduces direct competition to a minimum while permitting maximum parental investment (Sulloway, 1997). Diversification thus reduces competition, increases parental investment, and leads to children being less dependent on their parents.

Sulloway (1997) also examines the influence of birth order on sibling diversity.

- The firstborn tends to be advantaged and is the first to choose his niche within the family. This child tends to respect the status quo, to be socially authoritarian, and defensive in protecting his own interests, identifying him/herself more with the parents and to be both more jealous and more sure of himself.
- The middle child, in-between the other two, tends to look for new solutions to the family niche problem, making extreme or radical choices. This child may have recurring feelings of self-doubt

and be terrorized about getting lost in a "no-man's land" (Hug-Hellmuth, 1921).
- The youngest child has the greatest advantage from diversification and cultivates other abilities, thus reducing to a minimum confrontation (where he might be at a disadvantage compared to the others). This child tends to have an open mind, to be versatile, inventive, original, and attracted to new ideas and experiences.

* * *

We were amazed to note that even in this sextuplet group analogous factors of differentiation were at work, both in the mother's perceptions and the children's responses. Birth order, order of going home, weight, and sex made the children different from the very beginning. There were the two "firstborns" (Alice and Bruno), the "middle" children (Carlo and Daniele) and the "youngest" children (Elisa and Franco).

The two firstborns consider themselves, as much as is possible given this unique situation, the only children, and the mother seems to have greater expectations in their regard. Alice is a wilful and socially authoritarian child; Bruno, the most self-absorbed child, wants to please only his mother.

The middle children do not have an easy time finding their place in the family; the mother gives less time and attention to them and for various reasons her relationships with them are more difficult. Carlo is slower than the others in his psychophysical development; his behaviour indicates non-acceptance by the sibling group, and he manifests total intolerance of the situation by his continual temper tantrums. Daniele seems to live outside or at the edge of the group; he is very active and constantly in motion but goes unnoticed and is scarcely seen or heard.

The last two to be born (Elisa and Franco) are often less controlled by the mother and tend to be more open and interested in exploring their surroundings. They are the most adaptable and the more sociable children. Both have a close relationship with a substitute maternal figure. Different from the idealized children (Alice and Bruno) and the problem children (Carlo and Daniele), they both manage to cope on their own and to defend themselves openly, capable of healthy aggressiveness, and ready to fight for what they want.

Although the family was well organized to give the children the same experiences, from the outset distinct life events, inevitably, contributed to making them different. For example, Alice and Bruno, the first pair sent home from the hospital, were the only two who received breast feeding. Bruno was the only one of the boys not to have surgery as an infant for inguinal hernia. Franco was the only one of all the sextuplets to be sent back to the hospital after just a few days at home because he cried all the time. This particular circumstance altered the two-by-two schedule for sending the children home, and Carlo was thus the last to leave the hospital and alone rather than one of a pair.

The children reached the various stages of development at pretty much the same time and usually in the same order: the "firstborns" first, and then the others sometimes with major or minor difficulties. As in all families with many children, illnesses were passed from one to another, meaning that even a simple cold might take a few weeks to disappear from the household.

Sexual differences also had an influence. The two girls were able to distinguish themselves as individuals better than the four boys. The mother's relationship with the girls seems to have created a particular sub-group, similar to that of twins. Alice is considered the "bigger" sister and Elisa the "little" sister, and the mother attends to the older daughter and entrusts the younger one to the grandmother.

We hypothesize that the mother has a strong sense of identification with Alice, who was the firstborn girl, and has a decisive character just like her mother, who may have projected into this daughter her own childhood desire to be the firstborn rather than the middle child, "the shadow between two brothers", to quote from her book. Alice seems to be in unison with the mother's projected feelings and, apparently, to feel comfortable in this situation.

Elisa, a tiny delicate baby, was the second to last to be born, and immediately entrusted to grandmother's care. According to the mother, Elisa resembles her own younger brother and this might have stimulated in the mother unconscious feelings of jealousy and sibling rivalry. We wonder how the child herself experiences this projection. Further on Elisa shows a particular capacity for adaptation typical of the lastborn child (Sulloway, 1997; Piontelli, 1992). She also shows signs of a defensive mechanism individuated by Freud (1920, p. 153), that of "stepping aside" and "yielding the way" in favour of her "older" sister in the relationship with the mother. This he described as a fairly frequent phenomenon in sibling relationships whereby some siblings restrain themselves instead of competing with the other siblings, evidencing "very complicated psychic conditions". Notwithstanding this, Elisa does not renounce finding gratifying responses that satisfy her need for affection and exclusive care. For example, not only is she the grandmother's "pet", she is also the "darling" of a young adolescent girl who regularly comes to visit her in the family home.

Between these two sisters and the mother there seems to have been established that which Sharpe and Rosenblatt (1994) call a "sibling Oedipal triangle". These two authors maintain that sibling relationships develop autonomously and evolve structurally from a dyadic pre-Oedipal phase to a triadic Oedipal one. In families with more than one child, the children create triangles that are independent from the Oedipal parental triangles, which exercise a strong influence on psychic development. These sibling triangles can comprise two siblings and one parent, or three siblings, and they are based on ambivalent feelings that fluctuate between admiration and competition, submission and rebellion. We have seen in both Alice's and Elisa's profiles that this particular relational constellation, involving both of them and the mother, has influenced the development of the girls' personalities.

* * *

The subgroup of the male children comprises the firstborn of the boys (Bruno), the two middle children (Carlo and Daniele) and the lastborn child (Franco). The matriarchal family structure was without doubt an important factor in the development of the boys' personal identities and in their differentiation. In proportion, the father and the grandfather were less present in the sextuplets' daily life than the many female figures (mother, grandmother, various other carers), and they were subordinated to the mother's organization of the family that depended prevalently on assistance from the grandmother. Moreover, one must not ignore the fact that the media, with their repeated reportage focused on the "super" mother, had an effect on her. No one ever mentioned a "super" father!

It was above all on Bruno, the firstborn of the boys, into whom the mother seemed to project her own intellectual aspirations, as if she were assigning him a special, idealized role, different from that of the other male children in the family. We note that in an interview for a newspaper the mother calls him "the philosopher". This child, who was evaluated (at the neuromotor-relational examination in infancy) as "not very efficient in his postural and motor responses, but capable of showing attention to his surroundings", might have had an inborn gift of attentiveness to his environment which was probably reinforced by the mother who had strong intellectual expectations of him. Thus, he became a sensitive, thoughtful child who preferred to play by himself or with his sisters rather than with his brothers, and in so doing he avoided direct competition with the latter.

Carlo from the outset showed overall slower development than the other children, with whom he was unable to keep pace. He was not very active and paid little attention to his surroundings. He was often overcome by the others; they took his toys away or arrived ahead of him, and he reacted by throwing tantrums, without making himself understood. Reciprocal feelings of rejection were established between him and the others. The mother says that she cannot understand what he wants, and does not know how to help him. Carlo is the sextuplet who has the unrealistic desire to be an only child and receive all the mother's attention.

The mother calls Daniele an "active" child meaning that he is autonomous and independent, needing little or no care. He seems to be less present in her mind than the other children. He is always in motion, sometimes dangerously so, and prefers his own bodily sensations to the company of his brothers. Although he often prefers to play with his brother Franco, his relationships with the other siblings were generally transient, undifferentiated and not very affectionate.

The lastborn, Franco, seems freer from the mother's projections and expectations than the other boys. He is a lively and friendly child, interested in what his brothers are doing and willing to get involved and play with them. He gets along with everyone, in different ways and for varying amounts of time, depending on the situation. This flexibility in behaviour corresponds to his ability to be himself and express his feelings openly with both the mother and his brothers, in particular with Bruno and Carlo. He likes to be with his brothers (and also with the adults) as if an abundance of interpersonal relationships is for him an enrichment rather than a deprivation.

The father treats his four sons more or less in the same way, without differentiating them or demonstrating special affection. He gives each one his attention, leaving the initiative up to them, but he is always ready to intervene to set limits and see that everyone's rights are respected. He is available for one-to-one relationships and responds willingly to individual requests for help, or to play, or to be heard without being over-burdened by having to organize the group. The children return his affection and are very attentive to what he does and says, and they are quick to respect the few rules and limits that he sets. This situation shows that the father is capable of carrying out his paternal function by intervening with appropriate requests and actions.

Alice, the daughter who seeks out the father and requests his attention, and the one from whom he accepts and reciprocates such attention, gives him the satisfaction of an affectionate and playful father-daughter relationship.

The grandmother, a fundamental presence, notwithstanding the fact that she remains behind the scenes, is a guarantee of stability and nourishment, both physical and psychological, for the entire family. She seems capable of keeping in mind each of the children at every turn, paying attention to their individual needs, problems, and illnesses and, in so doing, performs a fundamental role in supporting her daughter's maternal function. Moreover, she takes upon herself the sleeping problems of the two "youngest" sextuplets, Elisa and Franco (see chapter II, paragraph 6). She also has a preferential relationship with her "pet" (Elisa), assigned to her from the very beginning by the mother.

* * *

Thus far we have described how the various circumstances and the household environment have had specific influences on each sextuplet, contributing to their different relationships with the adults and with each other. This helped each one to find its own niche, guaranteeing individual survival and healthy development.

When the sextuplets were three and a half years old, we were able to see that being in six had given them a good start and a solid foundation. The sextuplets seemed well on the way to structuring their individual personalities while being, at the same time, a strongly cohesive group. Conflict between the single child and the sibling group was minimal and at times completely absent.

This sextuplet group evidenced a strong feeling of an all-in-one family (Cierpka, 1993), a particular perception of unity that requires compromises to avoid the risk of destroying family unity. This means that individual interests take second place and family interests come first. For the most part we have observed a balanced and positive relationship between family functioning and the children's individual psychological evolution.

Lorenz (1935) observed that ducklings from the same family showed intense attachment to each other that did not exclude attachment to the parents. While still in the nest they recognized and understood each other: they showed solidarity and synchrony with each other in the sense that they ate and slept when they saw each other doing so. Being together was therefore a good beginning. But after having taken wing they no longer recognized each other and the so-called sibling understanding dissolved.

What will happen to our sextuplet group when the children are grown up and begin to take wing? Different from what happens in the animal world, separation from the family "nest" does not necessarily mean separation from the sibling group.

# CHAPTER FIVE

# Follow-up fifteen years later

Various follow-up encounters with the family took place in the period approximately 15 to 18 years after the end of the infant observation visits. Table 2 lists the encounters, specifying when they took place and the reason or type of contact; the tests administered were standard reactive tests and a socio-relational questionnaire and the contacts were limited to visits to the home and telephone conversations with the mother. First we present information regarding the home visits by using the observational method so as to bring the reader up to date on the sextuplets' development and important events that had taken place in their lives since the end of the infant observation (last observation at three years and six months).

## Three follow-up home visits

Three follow-up home visits took place at one-year intervals beginning approximately 15 years after the end of the three-year period of infant observation. It was evident that changes had gradually taken place in this lapse of time within the family, in particular in the sextuplet group. We noted certain specific traits for each individual

Table 2. Follow-up visits and psychological tests.

| Chronology (sextuplets' age) | Type of contact or test |
| --- | --- |
| 18 years, 2 months | Personality tests<br>Projective tests |
| 19 years, 4 months | WAIS<br>1st follow-up house visit |
| 20 years, 6 months | Socio-relational questionnaire<br>2nd follow-up house visit |
| 21 years, 6 months | 3rd follow up-house visit |
| 20–21 years | Telephone conversations<br>with the mother |

sextuplet in regard to psychosexual development, socialization, and study and work interests outside the family environment.

*First follow-up visit (19 years and four months)*

At the first follow-up visit the observer found all the family at home, except the father who was at work. The mother still played a central role. After gathering everyone in the living room she brought the observer up to date on the sextuplets. She did most of the talking and the others listened. Notwithstanding the inevitable physical development and changes that the six children had undergone since the time of the last infant observation, the observer had little trouble identifying them and recognizing in each sextuplet the child she had known 15 years before. They were all about the same height and were similar in build, and the observer had the impression that they were happy to be together. Also present was a taller male adolescent with a different physiognomy, who was introduced as a friend of Elisa's (similarly, as observed in infancy, Elisa had a "friend" who came to the house to be especially with her).

Some of the sextuplets greeted the observer with a smile, others gave no sign of recognition. The mother was pleasant and vivacious, as always. The grandmother had not changed much, but the grandfather was thinner and appeared to be in poor health.

Alice sat down on the floor next to the armchair where the mother was sitting and looking up to her listened attentively.

Bruno, the one whose physical looks had changed the most, went nervously back and forth between the kitchen and the living room.

Carlo stood facing the mother and next to Alice.

Daniele and Franco, who immediately decided to be the first two to take the test, went off to two different rooms with the two examiners.

Elisa sat down on the floor facing her mother, on the opposite side of the living room with her boyfriend at her side. A couple of times she went to sit on the arm of the grandmother's chair and they exchanged affectionate gestures. Her boyfriend appeared to be well integrated into the group.

When the first two finished the test, Alice offered to take her turn and the mother urged Carlo to do the test at the same time. Franco, who had just taken the test, gave Carlo an affectionate tap on the shoulder and told him not to worry because he, too, had not known how to answer some of the questions. Daniele appeared sulky and cross as he went into the kitchen without saying a word to anyone.

The mother accompanied the observer out onto the porch at the back of the house; the grandfather came too and talked nostalgically and at great length about the beautiful view of the countryside and how it had changed over the years.

At this point Daniele appeared and took over the conversation. He talked about himself and his community service work (a type of national service), commenting on and criticizing its disorganization. When the grandfather left, Daniele's conversation became a rather excited monologue that monopolized the observer's attention for some time. His discourse was interrupted when the mother and grandmother came and offered her something to drink. The mother mentioned that she is worried about Carlo and how the test was going.

When the second pair had finished the WAIS, Alice ran to join Franco who was with a friend from a nearby house. There were allusions indicating that he was Alice's boyfriend, but it was not stated explicitly.

Carlo went directly to the mother, who reassured him saying that the test went fine.

Then Bruno and Elisa, who were studying together in the dining room, went to take the test.

Both Carlo and Daniele remained in the house, each one on his own.

The mother stayed to talk for a while with the observer, especially about Carlo, who she thought had had difficulty with the test. Then, since it was getting late, she went to the kitchen to help the grandmother prepare dinner.

This visit evidenced certain aspects of continuity with the findings of the infant observations. Alice was the "top student" and the mother's alter ego. Elisa continued to be affectionately close to the grandmother and had a special relationship with someone outside the family circle (which reminds us of her childhood relationship with the adolescent girl who used to come and play with her). The mother's preoccupations about Carlo calls to mind a similar reaction she lived through when he did the Brunet-Lezine psychomotor test.

There were also evident signs of change. Both Alice and Elisa now had boyfriends, a common situation in adolescence, but this pointed out a difference between the two female and the four male sextuplets. Daniele, in the past, according to the observer's perception of him as the "forgotten" child, now showed an egocentric attitude and tried to attract the full attention of the observer. Bruno appeared anxious and uneasy, a bit on the sidelines, as if he could not find his place in the group.

## Second follow-up visit (20 years and six months)

During the telephone conversation to schedule the second follow-up visit, the mother announced the grandfather's death. When the observer arrived at the home, only the grandmother was there, preparing the meal as usual. She remarked that they had discovered that Carlo has the same kidney disease the grandfather had, only with onset at a much earlier age.

Bruno arrived soon after and showed off, telling the grandmother about his university studies. He then talked to Franco who was taking the final exams for his *Liceo*(secondary school) diploma. Daniele was also home, but upstairs sleeping. The other four were out; they had gone to a "rave" party the night before and had not yet returned home.

The mother arrived hot and angry because she had been informed that the cleaning lady was not coming. Her face was tired and showed signs of strain. After refreshing herself she answered the telephone and talked with a relative about the timing of an aunt's funeral. She explained to the observer that the other children were on their way home, as agreed. Alice, Elisa and Franco had taken Carlo with them to the night-time party.

The party group arrived one at a time. Carlo came in first, and went to the mother complaining of a headache. Alice was the only one to greet the observer with kisses on the cheeks and a handshake. Elisa gave a quick smile. Franco went to the kitchen to get something to eat. They began seating themselves around the table, waiting for Daniele to join them so that they could start filling out the socio-relational questionnaires. Daniele arrived soon after, his hair unkempt and his head between his shoulders; he sat down unwillingly without greeting anyone.

It took them about 20 minutes to do the questionnaire, after which they all got up and left and the mother gathered the papers with their answers and looked them over quickly, making a few corrections, just like a teacher.

After this the mother told the observer about some of her doubts and fears regarding the future. She now perceived her maternal role as precarious and, criticizing herself, added that due to life events and the children's attitudes, some of them no longer wanted a mother who was "commanding and intrusive". She gave merit to her husband as a parent and expressed her displeasure that the children had not chosen him more in the questionnaire. She also said that she was afraid of rivalry and jealousy among the sextuplets: "There are so many awful things on television." She felt guilty about Carlo's problems, and she reproached herself for certain choices made in the past about schooling. She felt threatened by the children's manifestations of autonomy and the impossibility of managing them all together as a group, which calls to mind the phrase in her book: "It was wonderful when I could feed them all at once with only one spoon" (see chapter II, paragraph 10).

This second visit was pervaded by an atmosphere of mourning; there was less family cohesion and there were signs of different prospects among the sextuplets. Carlo is the only one with a chronic illness. Three of the children, Alice, Bruno and Elisa, are enrolled at the university. Franco failed his final exams and had to repeat the last year of high school. Carlo and Daniele have interrupted their studies. Most of them are at ease and more or less relaxed, except for Carlo and Daniele who appear nervous, worried, and less well integrated. The group of sextuplets appeared to be divided between those who were projected outwards towards new relationships (Alice, Elisa and Franco) and those more withdrawn and solitary (Bruno, Carlo and Daniele).

### Third follow-up visit (21 years and six months)

None of the sextuplets was home at the third follow-up visit and the grandmother was about to go out with her brother to do the shopping. The mother complained about a backache. That morning she had slept late and she added, "That's not normal for me." She dramatically recounted the details about the death of the paternal grandfather, her father-in-law, who had recently been living with them. She then talked about the children, saying where they were and what they were doing.

Franco and Elisa were in Greece with their respective companions. Franco had a bad cold when they left.

Daniele went to work (a factory job) this morning, since he had woken up in a good mood.

Carlo was at the hospital for a treatment.

Bruno had gone alone to the family house at the beach.

Alice was working at a roadside restaurant, with her boyfriend.

The mother used her mobile phone to call the children, first Carlo and then Franco, saying that she was still a "mother hen" and too attached to the children. She was afraid she had made mistakes with them. Thinking about the past, she evaluated, like a teacher does, the consequences of the fact that when the sextuplets were children "It wasn't possible to stay indoors, so we always went out", and for that reason the children "never learnt to build towers or did puzzles, a game that requires concentration … and now they tend to be more interested in literary things than mathematics."

In addition to the pain of having lost her own father and that of the more recent death of her father-in-law, she now seems to fear separation from the children. Suddenly she turned away from such depressing thoughts and started to talk about her resentment towards the people who continued to accuse the family of "using public money", people who do not want to understand the many problems they have with so many children.

On this occasion the observer requested the consent of all the members of the family to publish the research project, and she asked the mother specific questions about her pregnancy and the first months following the birth. The mother answered willingly and before saying good-bye she spontaneously recounted a pleasant episode from her past. Once, in the summer, when she was with her father in a café, a young couple went by a few times and the young man kept pointing her out to his girlfriend. Her father then said, "Yes, this is my daughter who is the mother of the famous sextuplets." It was a memory of happy times, not only as a famous and admired super-mother, but also as the only daughter of her father.

This was the first time that the mother had been alone for such a long time with the observer. Encouraged by the questions asked, she talked openly about herself. She reviewed events and experiences of the infant observation period as if she were summing up her experiences as a young mother, giving this visit the feeling of leave-taking that had been missing many years earlier when the infant observations ended.

## Psycho-diagnostic tests

When the sextuplets turned 18 their paediatrician asked the parents' consent to give the children a series of tests to evaluate their cognitive, psychodynamic, and socio-relational development. The various tests were administered over a period of approximately three years and evidenced a specific pattern of evolution for each individual sextuplet.

- *Projective personality tests (18 years and two months)*

(administered and analyzed by Filippo Filippini, M.D., a medical psychologist)

The test was divided into two parts: two drawings and a written section. The written instructions were:

1. Draw your family
2. Draw your internal organs and describe what you have drawn
3. Write 10 lines about yourself and sign it at the end.

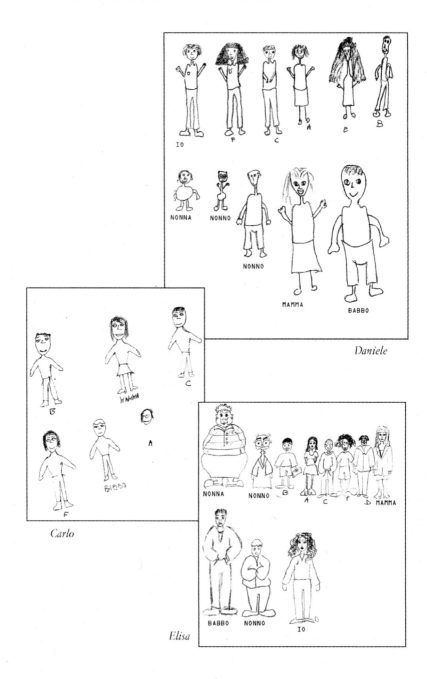

Daniele

Carlo

Elisa

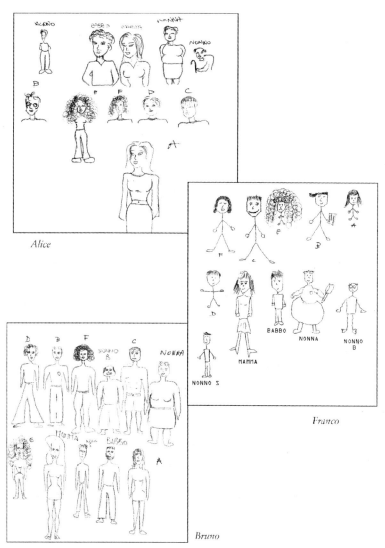

Alice

Franco

Bruno

IO = Me   A = Alice   B = Bruno   C = Carlo   D = Daniele   E = Elisa
F = Franco   MAMMA = Mommy   BABBO = Daddy   NONNA = Grandmother   NONNO = Grandfather

Figure 5.  Draw your family.

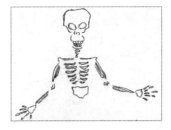

Alice: *This is the physical structure of my body from the head to the pelvis*

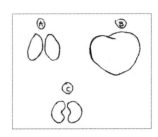

Elisa: *I have drawn:  A = lungs; B = heart; C = kidneys*

Carlo: *I have drawn a heart*

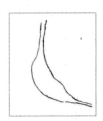

Bruno: *I have drawn my stomach*

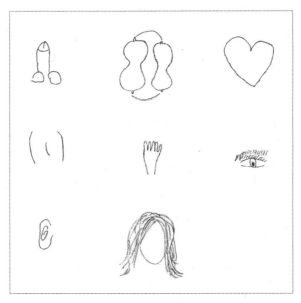

Daniele: *[left to right, top row]: penis, kidneys, heart
middle row: bottom, hand, eye
bottom row: ear  hair*

Our analyses of the family drawings (see Fig. 5) were based principally on Passi Tognazzo (1975), Corman (1967), and Tambelli,
Zavattini and Mossi (1995). At the time the paternal grandfather was
also part of the family, and all the sextuplets except one (Carlo) completed the drawing. None of the sextuplets eliminated him/herself
from the drawing. Not including oneself can signify maladjustment
within one's family or perception of oneself as not belonging to the
family (Passi Tognazzo, 1975). The names of all the persons represented are specified, written above or below each figure. All the sextuplets used the entire space available on the page, and the figures
are arranged more or less in two rows with the exception of one
drawing (Alice's). All sextuplets presented a personalized distribu-
tion of the family members, sometimes with humour (Elisa) and
placed their own figure in a distinct position in relation to the family group. The drawing ability is generally good and each drawing
shows a personal style.

Significant factors evaluated in the family drawings point to the
importance of specific family members (see the size of the figures)
and the affectionate ties existing among them (see where they are
placed in relation to one another). In addition the way the adult
couples (parents and grandparents) are drawn, side-by-side or separated, indicates a capacity, or lack thereof, to acknowledge adult
sexuality which is a fundamental part of the process of acquiring a
psycho-sexual identity in adolescence.

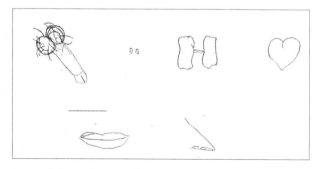

Franco: *[left to right, top row]: penis, kidneys, lungs, heart*
*bottom row: mouth, nose*

Figure 6. Draw your internal organs and write down a description of
what you have drawn.

The analysis of the results of internal organs drawings (Fig. 6) was based on symbolic meanings, given the lack of manuals with standardized evaluation processes, although we did refer to the Inside-of-the-Body-Test used by C.B. Tait and R.L. Ascher (1995), primarily for psychosomatic patients, and by Soifer (1985) for pregnant women.

All the self-presentations were written with personal and thoughtful remarks and different levels of introspection. The sextuplets mentioned specific characteristics of their own personalities and some made comments about their school life and their feelings about it. Two of the four boys mentioned their interest in sports (Daniele and Franco). Three of the six referred to their big family (Elisa, Daniele and Franco); the latter two specified having five siblings all their "same age".

Obviously there were differences in handwriting which were especially apparent in their individual signatures.

- *WAIS (19 years and four months)*

(administered by Angela Sforza and Mario Ruocco, both psychologists, and analyzed by the former)

Qualitative evaluation showed that all except one of the sextuplets (Carlo) had an average IQ, with slight variations depending on the verbal and non-verbal score ratios. The profiles of the various unelaborated scores were fairly similar. All the sextuplets' verbal scores were higher than their non-verbal scores. Certain differences between the sextuplets and specific individual personality characteristics were evidenced, especially regarding cognitive style, anxiety control and interest toward the outside world.

- *Socio-relational questionnaire (20 years and six months)*

(drawn up by Linda Root Fortini and Laura Mori, the authors, and analyzed by them)

The aim of the questionnaire was to evaluate the individual sextuplets' relationships within the family, including their siblings. The questionnaire was filled in at a single group sitting (during the second follow-up home visit), and covered three specific areas:

a. Relationships with the family adults in the past and at the present time (Table 3)

Table 3. Socio-relational questionnaire (Part a).

| Relationships with family adults (in the past and now) | | | |
|---|---|---|---|
| | *When you were little whom did you prefer to play with? Choose one: mother, father, grandmother, grandfather, others (specify)* | *When you were little whom did you turn to for help? Choose one: mother, father, grandmother, grandfather, others (specify)* | *Now whom do you turn to for help? Choose one: mother, father, grandmother, grandfather, others (specify)* |
| Alice | My brothers and sister | Mother/ Grandmother | Usually myself |
| Bruno | Mother | Mother | My best friends |
| Carlo | Mother | Mother | Father |
| Daniele | Others | Mother | Mother |
| Elisa | Brothers and sister | Mother | Boyfriend |
| Franco | Daniele | Mother | Mother |

b. Relationships with the other sextuplets in the past and at the present time (Figures 7 and 8)

c. Personal questions regarding how they imagined their future and considerations on living in a family as one of a group of sextuplets (Table 4).

Our analysis of the answers to item b (Figures 7 and 8) was based on the graphic representation created by Moreno (1964) for measuring social relationships. We decided to use this method notwithstanding the very small size of our sample because it allows visualization of the real positions of subjects in normal life situations. Moreno's explanation was: "The sociogram is a structural analysis of a group that allows measurement of the degree of organization in social groups [...] it studies the social structures in the light of the attractions and repulsions that are [manifested] within a group [...]. The greater the number of choices of reciprocal attraction, the higher the level of interest and participation within the group and, thus, the

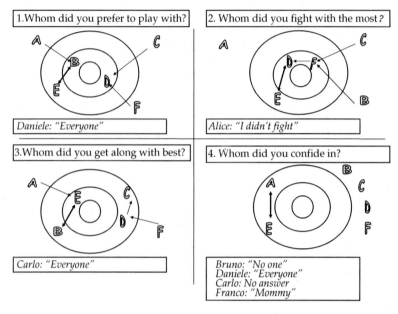

Figure 7. Socio-relational questionnaire (Part b-past)—Relationships with brothers and sisters in the past.

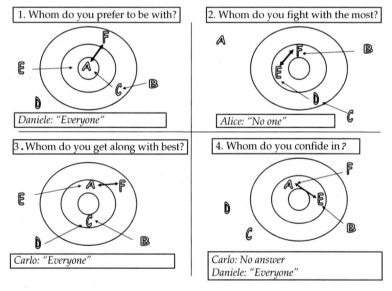

Figure 8. Socio-relational questionnaire (Part b-present)—Relationships with brothers and sisters now.

Table 4.  Socio-relational questionnaire (Part c).

| Prospects for the future | | | | |
|---|---|---|---|---|
| | *Thinking back to your childhood, what is your feeling about being a sextuplet? (Choose one: Easy, Complicated, Stimulating, Tiring, Positive, Negative)* | *Thinking about your future, what type of work would you like to do?* | *Where do you think you'll be living a few years from now?* | *Whom do you think you'll be living with a few years from now? (Choose one: with a friend, at home like now, other)* |
| Alice | positive | A worthwhile career in an artistic field | In the country, but near a city | With a friend |
| Bruno | positive | Accountant | [name of the provincial capital] | With a girl |
| Carlo | positive | School janitor | On my own | With a friend |
| Daniele | helpful | Millionaire | [name of their town] | With my girlfriend |
| Elisa | positive | I don't know | I don't know | With a friend |
| Franco | positive | In a creative/ alternative field | In a city | In the family I live with now |

greater the number of harmonious relationships. Instead, the greater the number of structures of isolation, the lower the level of interest and, thus, the greater the disorganization and lack of harmony."

## *Individual evaluations*

### ALICE

#### *Family drawing*

Alice drew herself in the foreground and larger than the other figures: indicative of aggressiveness and self-confidence (Passi Tognazzo,

1975). By placing herself alone in the foreground, she seems to express a feeling of self-importance as being the "firstborn", a role in synchrony with that chosen for her by the mother. There is a clear resemblance between her figure and the one representing the mother: the two are almost identical with accentuated female sexual characteristics.

She has divided the family into groups, with the adults above and the sextuplets below. The two couples (parents and grandparents) are represented in pairs.

All the figures are incomplete, including herself. She has drawn only the faces of her brothers; her sister is drawn with an almost complete body, from which the arms are missing. Omission of body parts signifies difficulty in making contact and conflicting feelings about one's sexuality (Passi Tognazzo, 1975).

## Internal organs drawing

She drew herself as a skeleton "from the head to the pelvis", evidencing the bone structure without reference to any internal body organs. This response to the instructions is original, but incongruous, as if the request had provoked some disturbance. Such a response is similar to the shock reply to table VII in the Rorschach test, the one commonly called the female or maternal table because it presents a concave form. How the subject interprets this table is generally considered to give an indication of the affective relationship with the mother in early infancy: the empty area in the centre of the figure may be disturbing for the subject, and such a reaction is evaluated as the "shock of emptiness". "A reaction of surprise is related to anxiety regarding sexuality, and in a woman this might mean refusal of femininity or sexuality" (Passi Tognazzo, 1979, p. 105).

## Written self-presentation

Alice introduced herself by writing her surname and then her first name; she wrote her age, followed by the words "even if I don't look it" (a typical sign of female vanity). She talks only about herself, with no mention of the family or the other sextuplets. By admitting to having had difficulty in making friends with her female peers, she seems to be aware of having some kind of problem relating to others. She claimed that she gave a lot to her friends, receiving little from them, but that she was anyway satisfied with the situation. She manifested indifference and slight scorn towards others and expressed the desire to live "by myself", admitting that it bothered her to think about the future.

## WAIS

She showed good cognitive abilities (abstraction, memory, attention). Her ability to control anxiety and to cope with new situations tended to vacillate when she was under stress. She also showed respect for social values, although she had a hidden tendency to oppose and criticize the outside world.

## Socio-relational questionnaire

a. She chose the mother as the person to whom she turned for help in the past, but declared she had no need of help from anyone at the present time and that she depended "generally on myself".
b. She answered that she had not fought with her siblings in the past, and that she did not fight with any of them even at the present. She indicated her brother Franco as the one whose company she preferred and with whom she got along best at the present time (his comments were reciprocal). She indicated her sister as her confidant both in the past and at present (Elisa's choices were reciprocal).

   There are noticeable differences between the responses to the questions regarding her relationships with her siblings in the past and the present. Alice was never chosen in answers referring to the past, but she was the one most chosen (three times) in reply to the question "Whom do you prefer to be with?"
c. Her answers to the questions about her future are clear, showing that she had aspirations for a career: she was the only one who said she would like to be a teacher (just like Mummy!), and preferences about where she wanted to live (in the country, but near a city, like her family).

## Closing analysis (Alice)

Alice showed a strong sense of identification with her mother and anxiety regarding the inside of her body, which calls to mind what

M. Klein (1932, p. 257) wrote about the psychosexual development of girls, characterized by a "primordial fear" that the inside of the body had deteriorated or been destroyed. Also Erikson (1968, p. 267) claims that the sense of the inner-bodily space is important in the female life cycle: "The female child [...] is disposed to observe evidence in older girls and women [of] the fact that an inner-bodily space—with productive as well as dangerous potentials—does exist. Here one thinks not only of pregnancy and childbirth, but also [...] all the richly convex parts of the female anatomy which suggest fullness, warmth, and generosity." In addition to the normal mother-daughter conflict, one must also keep in mind the fantasies that can be stimulated, in this particular situation, by her mother's exceptional pregnancy.

Thus, we note a marked discrepancy between outward signs of self-confidence and underlying anxiety related to her sexual body. Strong reciprocal mother-daughter identification during adolescence (already observed in infancy) increases the difficulties inherent in detachment and differentiation from the primary love object. Consequently, in her written self-presentation, Alice made specific references to her problem in establishing relationships with her female peers, as if it were difficult for her to find a new object of identification (that of a close friend).

This difficulty was evident also in her family relationships. For example, the family drawing reminds one of a family tree with a historical and hierarchical emphasis rather than based on affective relationships. The answers to the socio-relational questionnaire indicate that she is self-sufficient and is not involved with her siblings: she does not fight with them, neither now nor in the past. A discrepancy becomes evident when she claims to be detached from the sextuplet group at the present time, whereas the majority of her siblings have chosen her as the person to whom they would turn in case of need (as mother's carbon copy?).

## Bruno

### Family drawing

He placed himself between Daniele and Franco. This brotherly trio, all in a row and all the same height, forms a small sub-group. The figure of himself is the only one with a pocket where the heart is. Pockets are drawn by individuals dependent on the mother; when they are drawn on the chest they symbolize the breast, indicating feelings of oral and affective deprivation (Passi Tognazzo, 1975).

He gives importance to the mother; her figure is larger than all the others and he has placed it just below the figure representing himself.

The two couples, the parents and the grandparents, have both been separated by other figures. Moreover, the sextuplet group has also been divided, with the males in the upper row and the two females in the lower.

### Internal organs drawing

He drew only one organ, the stomach, with the entrance and exit canals, which calls to mind the function of nourishment that refers to the oral phase and the primary relationship with the mother.

### Written self-presentation

He began by writing only his first name and that he was "a fairly simple guy". Character-wise he described himself as "a bit of an introvert", adding that he liked animals a lot. He was happy with his studies and mentioned his decision to study business and economics at the university. He had a "passion" for music, especially singing (which had been observed in infancy). He wrote that he had few friends and did not go out with his peers.

### WAIS

His cognitive abilities are good and there were no signs of anxiety. He showed a remarkable degree of intellectual curiosity, few social interests, and scarce desire to compete with others.

### Socio-relational questionnaire

a. He had twice chosen the mother as the person to whom he turned in the past for help, but regarding the present his choice went outside the family to "my best friends".

b. He indicated Elisa three times as his favourite among the other sextuplets in the past (to which she reciprocated twice) and once as his confidant at the present (not reciprocated). In the past he had been chosen by both sisters as the sibling with whom they preferred to play, whereas at the present he was not chosen as the preferred one by any of the others.

c. He was the only one to indicate a specific future profession directly related to his university studies. He stated wanting to live in a city, probably with a girl, but near the family home so that he could visit often.

### Closing analysis (Bruno)

Both the family drawing and the internal organs drawing remind us of that little boy who wants to please his mother and has an infantile, almost fused, attachment to her.

In the self-presentation he described his feelings of isolation and being different from the rest of the sextuplet group, making one think that his drawing himself in the middle of the brotherly trio sub-group was the expression of a wish to reinforce his male identity. His answers to the socio-relational questionnaire evidence that Bruno is at the present marginalized within the sextuplet group: none of the other sextuplets ever referred to him in any of their choices. Instead, in the past, both sisters chose him twice as the one they preferred to play with as children, and he and Elisa chose each other also in answer to the question "Whom did you get along with best?", indicative of a particularly good feeling or affinity between them in childhood.

Bruno emphasized his university studies and his choice of a specific future professional identity that would help him feel integrated in the outside world with a good income and social status. Erikson (1968) believes that work goals, as concrete, practical activity corresponding with the requests of social reality, can strengthen the ego, support the repression of childish instincts, and reverse the tendency to passiveness.

In sum, this analysis recalls Meltzer's description (1979) of those adolescents who find it difficult to pass from a bisexual pubertal group mentality to that of heterosexual adolescents.

## Carlo

### Family drawing

His drawing is incomplete: he drew only six of the 11 family members. He was probably not able to finish in the time allotted.

He drew Bruno first and himself as the third figure, a position that can indicate self-depreciation (Passi Tognazzo, 1975).

He divided the parents, placing the mother as the centre figure of the three in the top row, and the father at the centre of the three in the bottom row, between Franco and Alice (incomplete figure). In this way he has represented a family of reduced dimensions, with a one-to-two parent-children ratio.

### Internal organs drawing

He drew only one organ, a heart, in the typical stylized form that symbolizes love, whereas the various small cracks drawn inside the perimeter suggest a broken heart (which calls to mind the mother's fantasy of foetal suffering in the first observation).

### Written self-presentation

He did not write either his given name or his surname. He wrote very few lines, all in block letters, with some spelling errors. He expressed his desire to be good at school and playing soccer.

### WAIS

The results indicated an overall intelligence deficit, in particular in regard to abstract thought. The examiner pointed out how much stimulation he had received from the family environment and added: "It is evident how much support his siblings gave him, reassuring him and minimizing the evaluative aspect of the test."

### Socio-relational questionnaire

a. He answered that as a baby he preferred to play with his mother and that he turned to her for help. He was the only one to indicate the father as the person to whom he turned for help at the present time.

b. The answers regarding his brothers and sisters are all generic ("everyone" or "no one") and are never reciprocated. He was chosen by others very few times. Bruno indicated him twice in questions regarding the present, and Daniele once, in answer to "Whom do you prefer to be with?" (not reciprocated).
c. He wrote that he wanted to become a school janitor, and that in a few years he would like to live on his own with a friend.

### Overall analysis (Carlo)

Albeit incomplete, his family drawing seems to represent his need for a more normal sized family with a lower parent-children ratio, which could mean not wanting to divide the parental care with so many siblings. This reminds us of his suffering as a child and his refusal of the group situation, which have continued. The drawing of the heart seems to be a graphic representation of feelings of deep pain related to his need to have a mother all for himself (observed also at nursery school, Chap II paragraph 12).

Notwithstanding the total lack of reciprocal choices with any of the other sextuplets in the answers to the socio-relational questionnaire, he appears to be accepted by them (see the WAIS examiner's comment, above). The developmental deficit, confirmed by the WAIS, has been compensated by the support given to him by all the other members of the family. As J. Dunn states (Dunn and Boer, 1992), the inadequacies of a sibling can induce greater involvement of the others, resulting in altruistic behaviour.

### Daniele

### Family drawing

He drew himself first, next to Franco: the two figures are almost identical, as if one were a mirror reflection of the other.

The sextuplets are all in the top row and the adults in the row below.

The two couples are drawn in pairs, but the parents are noticeably large, and the grandparents very small.

The father, the largest of all the figures, is represented as animated and smiling.

*Internal organs drawing*

He drew eight different body organs, filling up the entire page. First he drew a penis and two internal organs (kidneys and heart), then he continued with a series of external body parts (a bottom, a hand, an eye, an ear, and a head without facial features but with long hair) that may represent overwhelming and excitable sexual fantasies.

*Written self-presentation*

He introduced himself with only his first name, then his age, adding that he liked sports. He described himself as a "friendly" person who likes to be with others. He specified that he had a large family and a group of many siblings all his "same age". He was the only one to say that he did not want to continue studying, because he preferred going to work, and that he had chosen to do community work because he thought that "military service is a waste of time".

*WAIS*

The test showed that he had a more practical and concrete cognitive style rather than conceptual and/or abstract, as well as having a hyperactive tendency. He seemed more inclined to superficial interpersonal relationships but rather vulnerable when faced with situations that cause anxiety.

*Socio-relational questionnaire*

a. Although he did not choose an adult as the person he most wanted to play with as a child, twice he indicated his mother as the one to whom he turned for help, both in the past and at present.
b. His answers regarding his relationships with his siblings were all generic ("everyone"). Although he described himself as "friendly", none of the other sextuplets indicated him as their preferred companion at the present.
c. Regarding the choices for the future, he said that he wanted to be "a millionaire" and to live with "my girlfriend" in the town where the family lived.

*Overall analysis (Daniele)*

He described himself rather superficially in the self-presentation, and expressed vengeful and intolerable reactions towards the outside world although he defined himself as a "friendly" person. None of his siblings chose him as their favourite and his own answers about them were generic, indicating that he had no real preferences. His attitude about the future was based on an omnipotent fantasy of becoming a "millionaire".

Analysis of the results of the WAIS test reconfirmed his tendency to hyperactivity, which had been observed in childhood (including the constant sucking on a dummy).

The figures in the internal organs drawing evidence an altered mental representation of his own body. This leads us to think that there may have been developmental difficulties relating to the lack of integration of sexual body images and impulses with a proliferation of masturbatory fantasies, which calls to mind the question of identity confusion in adolescence, first studied by Erikson, who talked about identity diffusion in adolescence in reference to situations where the individual has split self-images and there is a "loss of centre" (Erikson, p. 212). Sexual impulses originating in the body are experienced as threatening and are neither held at bay nor integrated, indicating failure of the central masturbatory fantasy (Laufer, 1976).

The fact that he drew himself next to his brother Franco and that the two figures have a strong resemblance are a reminder of their close relationship in childhood and could indicate a deeper need in Daniele to define and reinforce his identity by using his twin brother Franco as his double ("soul mate", in Italian *"anima gemella"*) (Jeammet, 1992, p. 27), a fantasy frequently seen in siblings and characterized by complementary or parasitic ties rather than a symbiotic one, inasmuch as one of them is usually much more dependent than the other.

Daniele seemed to be experiencing what is commonly known as adolescent confusion about not wanting to grow up, that is related in part to the problems of dependence on parental figures and characterized by a mental state of pseudo-maturity, typical of those who are overly active in order to get on in the outside world (Meltzer, 1979).

*Elisa*

*Family drawing*

Elisa showed a sure hand and good drawing ability, characterizing almost all the family figures with humour and originality.

She drew herself apart from the rest of the sextuplet group and larger than her siblings and her mother, similar to how Alice drew herself.

The first row begins with a large, fat figure of the grandmother (which immediately catches the eye), followed by all the siblings, and ends with a relatively small figure of the mother (somewhat devalued as compared with the grandmother's). The lower row contains a large figure representing the father and, next to him, the paternal grandfather followed by Elisa herself wearing trousers, whereas both her mother and sister are depicted wearing skirts. The father and grandfather are drawn with a weaker and uncertain touch, indicative of shyness according to Passi Tognazzo (1975). Positioning herself next to the parent of the opposite sex could indicate a situation of Oedipal desire (Passi Tognazzo, 1975) that reminds us of the lack of a privileged relationship with the father during childhood.

She divided the parental couple, but drew her grandparents side-by-side (another sign of conflict with the mother).

*Internal organs drawing*

She drew three internal organs in the following order: the lungs, a heart, and the kidneys. The two double organs are small compared to the heart and almost symmetrical. This configuration reminds us of an Oedipal sibling triangle: a "mother" organ divided between two "sister" organs (see chapter IV, paragraph 4).

*Written self-presentation*

She introduced herself with her first and then her surname, specified where she lived and said that she was part of a large family. She said that she had always done very well at school but that this year she felt stressed. Now she hated school, did not like the subjects and considered the teachers "stupid". She even thought she had chosen the wrong school. She seemed to use the self-presentation as an opportunity to express anger and disappointment.

## WAIS

Analysis of the test results evidenced good judgment, concentration, sense of reality, ability for synthesis, and adequate anxiety control. The examiner commented that some of the questions were answered with "I don't know", indicative of a way of coping to avoid taking risks.

## Socio-relational questionnaire

a. Although she chose the mother as the figure of reference in the past, she was the only one to make a clear choice of a friend at the present.
b. She is the sibling with the greatest number of reciprocal choices (six times) regarding relationships with the other sextuplets. The only two non-reciprocal choices involve Alice for the two present time questions "Whom do you prefer to be with?" and "Whom do you get along with best?" In childhood she preferred to play with and got along best with Bruno, and she fought mostly with Daniele; for the present she said she fought with Franco. In both the past and present she chose her sister as her confidant: these two choices were reciprocal and indicate a special dynamic relationship between the two sisters.
c. Regarding the future she emphasized the importance of living with a friend. She gave two "I don't know" answers (as in the WAIS) to questions as to what kind of work she wanted to do and where she wanted to live in the future.

## Overall analysis (Elisa)

Her family drawing reconfirmed both a close bond with the grandmother and a conflict with the mother (observed in childhood). There was also evidence of another important relationship, the one with the sister (drawn vertically above her) and characterized by ambivalence: her sister seems to be a kind of double with whom Elisa can identify and from whom she can also differentiate herself.

The drawing of the two mirror-like images of double internal organs may illustrate the feeling of being part of a pair of twins and separate from the other four brothers. The large heart drawn between the two double organs could represent a sibling Oedipal triangle between the two girl "twins" and their mother. Herein a parallel conflict between two contrasting maternal images is graphically depicted: a particular situation in which the mother is either the symbiotic object contested by her two daughters or the disturbing element in a symbiotic–like relationship between the two sisters (Athanassiou, 1986).

Although, like Alice, she drew herself separate from the rest of the group of sextuplets, she did place herself in a position indicating more involvement with them.

In the written self-presentation strong feelings of displaced anger and hostility directed towards the outside world, represented by her school experience, clearly emerge.

The WAIS evidenced "excellent achievement" and the family drawing showed that she was good at drawing her family and had a good sense of humour. According to Freud, a good sense of humour is often used as a defence against painful affects (which involve limiting competition with her sister).

## Franco

### Family drawing

Franco drew himself first and in the top row, followed by his siblings.

In the bottom row he drew his parents and grandparents, as couples.

The faces of his siblings are expressive and well differentiated, but the bodies, all the same, minimized, and stereotyped, indicate childishness (Passi Tognazzo, 1975). The bodies of the adults are complete, more detailed and personalized.

The figures are done with a light touch denoting a refined character and delicate feelings (Corman, 1967).

### Internal organs drawing

He drew six body parts: three internal organs (kidneys, lungs and heart) and three external parts (penis, mouth and nose). The first figure is the penis, drawn with a firm stroke and obliquely, almost in line with the profile of the nose just below. Overall, the drawing seems to emphasize his male sexual identity.

## Written self-presentation

He introduced himself with his first name, stating his age and where he lived. He then wrote that he was a year behind at school because he had failed, an episode that differentiated him from the rest of the group. He mentioned that he had five siblings, all his "same age". He described himself as a person who was "timid, generous, nice to be with and very, very nervous", and stated categorically that "When I don't like something I suppress it 100% and totally disapprove of it" (showing an awareness of neurotic conflicts).

He wrote that he got along well with his friends and was closely "tied to the family", thus pointing out how important affectionate bonds were for him.

## WAIS

His good cognitive abilities were characterized by meticulousness and a tendency to lose himself in details rather than considering the overall position. The results evidenced generosity and a willingness to help others.

## Socio-relational questionnaire

Overall the answers to the questionnaire show remarkable internal coherence regarding affectionate bonds.

a. He specified the mother as the figure of reference both in the past and for the present, and as his confidant in the past.
b. Three times he named Daniele as his favourite companion from among the other sextuplets in the past, and the brother he got along with best, as well as the one with whom he quarreled most. He chose Alice twice in regard to the present, as the sibling he preferred to be with and the one he got along with best (she reciprocated these choices). And he specified that Elisa was the sibling he fought with most in the present (and she reciprocated this choice).

c. Although he did not name any specific preferences for his future, he did mention wanting to work in a "creative, artistic" field, an idea that proves coherent with his future choice of university studies. It appeared to be more important with whom he would live ("the family I live with now") than where, confirming the importance of his affectionate ties to others.

## Overall analysis (Franco)

In his written self-presentation Franco made a detailed, personalized self-portrait that shows good introspection. In the family drawing he drew himself first, thus indicating self-esteem, and gave particular importance to the mother (by drawing her larger than all the other figures, as Elisa did with the grandmother's figure), indicative of a good relationship. The internal organs drawing evidences that he had achieved a sufficiently integrated sexual body image.

He has a realistic perception of himself, that includes his limits and potential, with some discrepancies between his self-esteem and the esteem that others have of him, which could indicate a certain capacity for painful self-awareness. His generosity and willingness to help others, evidenced by the WAIS, also emerged in his self-presentation as well as in his behaviour towards his siblings, and appear to be related to an ability to put himself in other people's shoes.

He made an explicit differentiation between the sibling group, whose bodies are all depicted schematically in an extremely childish manner (Passi Tognazzo, 1975), and the adult group, whose bodies are more structured. This comparison would appear to indicate awareness of dependence and the ability to elaborate the depressive position during adolescence.

We are reminded of Meltzer's description (1979) of the adolescent as a person looking for a way to go forward towards a strong, independent adulthood while also looking back to being a child in the family. This backward and forward movement between different states of mind allows the adolescent to experiment being alone as well as keeping him in contact with the adolescent community. For Franco the way forward is marked by both self-esteem and the achievement of a psychosexual identity, together with receptive, sensitive aspects, such as altruism, worrying about others and an artistic inclination.

## Continuity and discontinuity in the sextuplets' development

We now wish to examine the elements of continuity and discontinuity in the sextuplets' development and to compare them with the childhood psychodynamic profiles. In commenting on their development in the period from ages 19 to 21 years, we focus on the problem of identity in regard to both consolidation of psychosexual development and subjective experience of the self. The evolutional process of identity acquisition implies individuation of a subjective self with perception of the continuity of one's own existence in time and space and an external self constructed through socialization and recognition from others.

The list of the sextuplets' important life events in the period specified (Table 5) focused on

- scholastic/occupational situation, as an index of integration with the outside world
- sentimental relationships, as an index of ability to achieve a psychosexual identity
- the 21st summer time activity, as an index of sociability and autonomy
- physical health and/or psychological problems.

Considering physical growth and appearance, the observer noticed during the follow-up home visits that the sextuplets were very similar in height and size. They had pleasant, harmonious features, but were all different notwithstanding family resemblance: some looked more like the mother, some the father, and some a combination of both.

An auxological study (*Il Nuovo*, 1999) showed that they were slightly lower than average in height compared to the reference population, with a variation among them less than that found among non-twin/triplet siblings. Their height graphs showed a take-off during the latency period: between the ages of seven and eight and a half years of age for the girls, and between eight and nine for the boys. This finding is not concordant with the graph for the reference population, where the height growth take-off normally occurs later, in adolescence. There was a slow-down of growth speed after the latency period, followed by delayed pubertal development in all six children. Thus, there was a dissociation between the age of peak in

Table 5. Life events in late adolescence.

|  | Occupation (work/study) | Sentimental relationships | Summertime activity at 21 years | Health constraints |
|---|---|---|---|---|
| Alice | University | Yes | Part-time summer job with boyfriend | Menstrual cramps |
| Bruno | University | Not reported, neither by him nor the family | Alone at the beach (family house) | /// |
| Carlo | Occupational school | No | At home for health reasons | Chronic renal insufficiency |
| Daniele | Community service (studies interrupted) | Yes, stormy and unstable | Took a job, but left it soon after | Developmental crisis |
| Elisa | University | Yes | Travel abroad with Franco and their respective partners | /// |
| Franco | University (after repeating last year of high school) | Yes | Travel abroad with Elisa and their respective partners | Gastritis |

the growth of stature and that of manifested sexual characteristics. This unusual growth curve has a curious implication: had Mother Nature intended to slow down what could have been an explosive six-fold impact of pubertal transformations in these siblings?

Longitudinal studies on low birth weight babies show that only a low percentage (25%) go to university and only 50% reach an average

IQ (see the research by Maureen Hack of Case Western Research University of Cleveland, OH, *New England Journal of Medicine*, 2001.)

The good psycho-motor development of our sextuplets (except for one) was first demonstrated by the Brunet-Lezine test (at 14 months and 12 days); it continued into adolescence, with WAIS scores of more than 100 for five of them, and was later reconfirmed by the fact that four of the six attended university. (At the end of the follow-up, when they were 25, two had university degrees, two were completing their university studies, and one was in occupational school.) Based on comparison of these data with the statistics reported above, and considering the results of the tests administered in childhood and late adolescence, the sextuplets classify as above average in intelligence.

This positive finding can be related to two different factors. First, the good medical assistance and, second, the mother's determination which permitted continuation of the pregnancy for as long as possible, with birth in the 34th week, meaning that the newborns did not need to be put in intensive care. International research done online by MOST (mothers of super twins) showed that the average length of pregnancy was 29 weeks in seven cases of sextuplets born in 1995. Thus, 34½ was a good start. Then, equally important, was the very favourable family environment with adults capable of organizing the home to cope with and give good care to the children, establishing affectionate relationships with the sextuplets as a group and, individually differentiated, with each one.

\*\*\*

As for their health, four of the sextuplets continued to be in good health while two had experienced conditions that differentiated them from the others: these were the two middle children, the ones who had had the hardest time finding their own niche within the family (see chapter IV, paragraph 4).

Carlo, the sextuplet who had already experienced more difficulties than all the others, developed in late adolescence a chronic kidney disease with important repercussions that risked increasing the discrepancy between him and all the others. It is well known that the onset of a physical disease in adolescence has a particularly great impact; it can disturb development, especially the individual's feelings of integrity and self-esteem, leading to regression and increased dependence, which in turn may create difficulties in identification with one's peers (Schowalter, 1983). This reminds us of the observer's original perception of Carlo as a "damaged child ".

Daniele in this period experienced psychological difficulties, which appeared shortly after two dramatic events: the death of the sextuplets' maternal grandfather and that of a friend. These deaths could have re-awakened threatening echoes of internal loss of the self. He interrupted his studies, had trouble holding down a job, and withdrew from his siblings and friends. The observer had noticed his personality change during the second follow-up home visit, when he subjected her to a long vindictive monologue and evidenced omnipotent behaviour. This situation has been resolved by psychoactive medicine and psychotherapy, a treatment that he and the family accepted, because they were all aware of the fact that he had problems. This developmental crisis is probably related to a disturbance that was already present in the earliest phase of his development, which has been evidenced in his psychodynamic profile. Thus, Daniele, "the forgotten child", is now one of his mother's major preoccupations.

The other sextuplets do not all have the same reactions to Carlo and Daniele. The follow-up home visits showed that the group (in particular Franco, at the time of the WAIS test) had an affectionate protective attitude toward Carlo. Another example is when they invite him to come along to the "rave" party. However, during childhood we observed mutual exclusion between him and the other sextuplets: they rarely if ever played together.

The answers to the socio-relational questionnaire show that although there are no reciprocal responses between Carlo and any of the others, his siblings now feel a certain amount of responsibility for him and take care of him. They treat him more as a younger brother than as a peer which seems to have been a helpful attitude that compensates for his inadequacies. Although Carlo's chronic physical disease differentiates him from his siblings it also stimulated their desire to help him and eventually their ability to understand him better. This positive attitude on their part has been an important sign of affection for all the siblings because it means sharing real emotional problems and dividing the task of taking care of a brother, rather than having to bear alone the heavy burden of a sibling with difficulties, as occurs in families with only one other child.

About Daniele's problem, conversely, his siblings seem to feel less comfortable, rather disoriented, and tend to keep their distance. This suggests that a psychological disorder may be more mysterious and threatening as well as misunderstood; thus it might well represent a situation that is potentially disturbing, destructive, and destabilizing for the group, because of "the fear of madness that is within us all" (Money Kyrle in *On the Fear of Insanity*, 1969).

\*\*\*

The two "firstborns" followed a linear development. The mother continued to be somewhat demanding of them in their late adolescence; she had great expectations and aspirations for them. These two were both conditioned by the mother's projections and their roles were fixed. Erikson (1968) referred to role fixation to indicate the difficulty a child had in undertaking free initiatives, in experimenting different roles spontaneously, and thus in experiencing more flexible personal relationships.

Alice appeared to be the big sister who stood in for the mother, demonstrating strong individualism. The fact that she was the one chosen the most times in the socio-relational questionnaire indicates general recognition of this role. Bruno, the most successful student of the brothers and the first to attend university, along with his sisters, has had difficulties in expressing his psycho-sexual identity which seems to have been concealed behind the role of an intellectual. In assuming this self-appointed label he distinguished himself from the others, remaining somewhat hidden and living at the edge of the group.

\*\*\*

Comparing the adolescent and the childhood profiles, we found overall more elements of continuity and cohesion than of discontinuity and disgregation in both the development of the individual sextuplets and their group relationships. At the time of the last contact the sextuplets had not yet made their definitive life choices; rather, they were at the beginning of the period called prolonged adolescence: manifestations of elements of discontinuity may yet occur before they reach full adulthood. Their different personalities, so distinct from each other, appeared constant even after the transformations of adolescence.

This sextuplet sibling group has remained united and continues to be characterized by a lack of rivalry and strong aggressiveness among themselves. It has not functioned as a closed enclave or as a clan to strengthen identity, or as a gang opposed to the outside world. Rather, the group appears to function like a community solidified over time through gradual elaboration of the dramatic impact of their birth as a group of sextuplets. This community seems to have nurtured its members and given them sufficient freedom of movement.

It appears that in adolescence this sextuplet sibling group was supportive, contributed to each sibling's sense of personal identity, and helped to contain difficult situations which might have resulted in potential regression.

We believe that it also carried out a function similar to that of a peer group which, through mutual recognition, permits individuals to distinguish themselves from adults without the need to break off ties or commit rebellious acts while protecting and consolidating self development. It is still too soon to evaluate how this sextuplet group will function in the passage to adulthood.

We think that P. Coles' query (2003) about identification processes—if there is a need or impulse to overcome and abandon sibling bonds similar to that aimed at resolving the Oedipal conflict and distance oneself from one's parents—is particularly significant for this sibling group of sextuplets who have grown up together in the same family environment for more than 20 years.

# CLOSING COMMENTS

The principal aim of this book is to study the evolution of a group of six same-age siblings and how this unusual experience influenced the development of each individual child and contributed to the construction of his/her personal identity. We have shown the continuity of relationships from childhood through late adolescence, an aspect of developmental psychology that has not as yet been sufficiently investigated in depth.

This sibling bond among the sextuplets, like the bond between a mother and the foetus-baby that is established before birth, has its origin in a biochemical, neurophysiological, and psychological union.

For the sextuplets, birth meant, as well as the loss of the intra-uterine environment, a separation from each other.

We have hypothesized that the constellation of relationships among multiple-birth children from triplets to sextuplets is different from that between twins and that, in addition to a primary need for attachment to the mother and the other same-age siblings, there is also a primitive need to feel part of a group. Just as the attachment to the mother has a biological basis, their sense of companionship is based on the primitive animal need for physical warmth (Bowlby, 1969).

Analogous to what happens with nestlings or a litter of puppies or kittens, the sextuplets shared evolutional intimacy and synchronic needs: they all "required the same part of the same thing at the same time" (Bourguignon, 2003). This is a primitive group function, similar to that observed in early mother-child interactions based on affective synchrony, imitation and non-verbal communication.

Each sextuplet's need for attachment and desire for intimacy and exclusive nurturing is inevitably frustrated, although compensated and satisfied by the sibling group that provides a different type of warmth, closeness, and security, and that in time becomes an environment of solidarity, sharing, and reciprocal teaching. The sibling group is, thus, just as much the original source of affection as the parents. "One can affirm the existence of an affectionate nucleus based on self experience that provides both a sense of continuity throughout evolutional change and a sense of empathy towards others"(Emde, 1989, p. 56).

After birth and going home, the sextuplets' experience of life together and belonging to a homogeneous group began once again. The mother's attitude (and that of the entire family) contributed to reinforcing the cohesion of the group, organizing it while diversifying each child. The mother used her professional identity as a teacher to cope with her six children all the same age, respecting their individual personalities and giving each one a place within the "group-class". While trying to be as fair as possible to each child, she promoted a "community feeling" that comes with the experience of fair and equal treatment for all, a need that lies at the base of human society and can be promoted by fraternal identification (Freud, 1921).

Faced with the mother's need to not be emotionally involved with her children (a defensive reaction to the painful part of being a mother), the children adapted and learned self-imposed limitations early in life: they respected the rules, did not ask for more than their due, and rarely fought with each other for any length of time. As observed during their childhood, their lack of aggressiveness had a "cushion effect" on their relationships with each other.

In addition to the mother-child relationship, the sibling relationship was fundamental in providing a healthy space for growth that helped them to live together, to form affectionate ties, and to feel comfortable in a group situation and not only in the intimacy and uniqueness of the mother-child relationship. Paradoxically, it was precisely the sextuplet group that on particular occasions provided the protection and affectionate support necessary for individual achievement during the various evolutional stages.

This unusual experience of being six siblings of the same age contributed, through an identification process, to the development of a "sense of us": that forgotten area in emotional development (Emde, 1983) which helps one distinguish affectively between himself and the other, between what can be shared and what cannot. The experience of having "many varieties of us" (Dalal, 1998) contributed to the sextuplets' experience of a wide range of different ways of relating to others—from that of inducting reciprocal processes of differentiation (niches) to that of developing their ability to establish early significant relationships among themselves in addition to those with the adults.

In Bossard's and Boll's (1956) research on large families, some of the responses of adults interviewed demonstrated that living in a large family helps one to learn at an early age that there are other people in the world and that, although privacy is often rare or almost non-existent, one acquires a vital group spirit that implies thinking and resolving things together. Moreover, in the give and take of everyday life, each person must learn to control his own emotions and to think in terms of "us" rather than "me" (Dunn, 1985, p. 90–91).

The group of sextuplets was still cohesive in late adolescence, able to adjust and adapt according to their individual needs and personal likes or dislikes, without isolating or expelling those siblings who manifested some difficulties; under certain circumstances, it functioned like an authentic adolescent peer group.

We verified the structural value of this experience in the social and psycho-affective development of the individual sextuplets. Our findings agree with current studies according to which sibling relationships can supply psychic nourishment and contribute to development in ways quite different from those of child-parent relationships. Therefore, they are not simply "secondary editions" of the Oedipal situation in that love and collaboration between siblings are not only reactive manifestations to rivalry and jealousy.

The question of bonds and relationships between the sextuplets in adulthood remains open. What influence will life events and individual choices have on belonging to a sextuplet group? Also, will their ability to develop exogamous ties be influenced by their particular childhood experience characterized by intermittent relationships with the mother, by a number of substitute carers, and by being a sibling group that supplies its own affection, protection, and understanding?

This study is based on the observation of early child development and family relationships in an exceptional sibling group of sextuplets. We have shown how the interaction between maternal attitude and the personal characteristics of each sextuplet influences individual personality development, hence confirming the uniqueness of each mother-baby relationship. We have also briefly discussed how the grandmother, an ever-present supporting figure, helps integrate essential aspects of maternal care while the father, a gentle and affectionate though peripheral parent during the first year of the children's lives, is a figure linked to different Oedipal experiences (observed especially in relation to his two daughters), and to the acquisition of distinct psycho-sexual identity (see the profiles of his four sons in late adolescence).

In the mind of each sextuplet, the group appears to have functioned as a basis for a sense of community, a supportive experience that contributed, in particular ways, and at different moments, to self-esteem, social adaptation and, at times, even to feelings of exclusion.

In this project Esther Bick's *Infant Observation* methodology has been used as a research tool to study a most unusual sibling group characterized by the fact that six siblings of the same age have lived together in the same family environment from infancy to adulthood. The development of these children's behavioural patterns in infancy and the mother-baby-group relationships have been observed in detail and longitudinally for a three-year period. The follow-up has revealed a greater continuity of development than discontinuity, which suggests once again that early detection of childhood difficulties might serve to prevent more complex problems in later development.

# REFERENCES

Algini, M.L. (Ed.) (2003). *Fratelli*, In: "Quaderni di Psicoterapia infantile—Nuova Serie", 47.

Athanassiou, C. (1986). *A study of the vicissitudes of identification in twins.* In: "Int. J. Psycho-Anal.", 67, 329–335.

Bank, S. & Kahn, M.D. (1982). *The Sibling Bond.* New York. Basic Books.

Battaglia, G. et al. (1982). *The Florence sextuplets. Report of a case. Part two: Progression of the onset of labor and delivery.* In: "Acta Europea Fertlitatis", vol. 13, n. 1, 25–34.

Bettelheim, B. (1969). *The Children of the Dream.* New York. Macmillan.

Bick, E. (1964). *Notes on infant observation in psychoanalytic training.* In: "Int. J. Psycho-Anal", 45: 558–566.

Bick, E. (1968). *The experience of the skin in early object relations.* In: "Int. J. Psycho-Anal", 49: 484–486.

Bion, W.R. (1961). *Experiences in Groups and Other Papers.* London. Tavistock Publications.

Bossard, J. & Boll, E. (1956). *The Large Family System.* University of Pennsylvania Press.

133

Bourguiron, O. (2001). *Complesso fraterno e socialità umana*, In: Algini M.L. (Ed.) (2003), *Fratelli* cit., 98–107.

Bowlby, J. (1969). *Attachment and Loss*, vol. I, London. Hogarth Press.

Bowlby, J. (1988). *A Secure Base: Clinical Applications of Attachment Theory.* London. Routledge.

Brazelton, T.B. & Cramer, B.G. (1991). *The Earliest Relationship.* London. Karnac Books.

Brunori, L. (1996). *Gruppo di fratelli. Fratelli di gruppo.* Roma. Borla.

Bühler, Ch. (1930). *The First Year of Life.* New York. John Day Co.

Bydlowski, M. (1997). *Il debito di vita: itinerari di filiazione.* Urbino. Quattro Venti. 2000.

Bydlowski, M. et al. (1991). *Maternal reactions to the birth of triplets.* In: "Acta Geneticae Medicae Gemmellologiae", 17, 453–460.

Cierpka, M. (1993). *Lo sviluppo del "sentimento familiare".* In: "Interazioni", 2, 11–28.

Coles, P. (2003). *The Importance of Sibling Relationships in Psychoanalysis.* London. Karnac.

Cooper, H. & Magagna, J. (2005). *The origins of self-esteem in infancy*, In: Magagna, J. et al. (Ed.), *Intimate Transformations.* London. Karnac.

Corman, L. (1967), *Il Disegno della Famiglia*, Bollati Boringhieri, Torino, 1970.

Dalal, F. (1998). *Taking the Group Seriously.* London. Jessica Lingsley.

Donzelli, Giampaolo et alii (1981). *The History of the Florentine Sextuplets: obstetric and genetic considerations*, In: "Prog Clin Biol Res.", 69A, 217–220.

Dunn, J. (1985). *Sisters and brothers.* London. Fontana paperback.

Dunn, J. & Boer, F. (Ed.) (1992). *Children Sibling Relationship: developmental and clinical issues*, New Jersey & London, Lawrence Earlbaum Associates.

Dunn, J. & Kendrick, C. (1982). *Siblings: Love, Envy and Understanding*, Cambridge Mass, Harvard University Press.

Dunn, J. & Plomin, R. (1990). *Separate Lives: Why Siblings are so Different*, Basic Books, New York.

Emde, R.N. (1983). *The prerepresentational Self and its affective care*, In: "The Psychoanalytic Study of the Child", 38, 165–192.

Emde, R.N. & Sameroff, A.J. (Ed.) (1989). *Relationship disturbances in early childhood: a developmental approach.* New York. Basic Books.

Erikson, E.H. (1968). *Identity Youth and Crisis.* New York. W.W. Norton.

Fairbairn, W.D. (1952). *Psychoanalytic Studies of the Personality*. London. Tavistock Publications Limited.

Ferrara Mori, G. (1984). *La metodologia dell'osservazione diretta della relazione madre-bambino e l'individuazione di precoci disturbi dello sviluppo emotivo*, In: "Acta Medica Auxologica", vol. 16, 135–137.

Fraiberg, S. (1982). *Pathological defenses in infancy*. In: "The Psychoanalytic Quarterly", L1, 612–635.

Freud, A. & Dann, S. (1951), *An experiment in upbringing*. In: "The Psychoanalytic Study of the Child", 6: 127–168.

Freud, S. (1905). *Jokes and their Relation to the Unconscious*, SE, VIII.

Freud, S. (1920). *The Psychogenesis of a Case of Homosexuality in a Woman*, SE, XVIII.

Freud, S. (1921). *Group Psychology and the Analysis of the Ego*, SE, XVIII.

Gaddini, E. (1974). *Sulla Imitazione*, In: *Scritti*, Milano, Cortina.

Garel, M. et al. (1994). *Two-year follow-up cohort studies on triplets: development of children and mother-child relationship*, In: "Arch. Pediatr.", 1(9), 806–812.

Garel, M. et al. (1997). *Psychological consequences of having triplets. A four-year follow-up study*, In: "Fertil. Steril.", 6, 1162–1165.

Garel, M. et al. (2000). *Les mères de triplés et leurs enfants. Evolution de 4 à 7 ans après la naissance*, In: "Gynécol Obstet Fertil", 28, 792–797.

Goshen-Gottstein, E.R. (1980). *The mothering of twins, triplets and quadruplets*, In: "Psychiatry", 43, 189–204.

Harris, M. (1987). *Towards learning from experience in infancy and childhood*, In: Harris Williams M. (Ed.), *Collected papers of Martha Harris and Esther Bick*, Perthshire, Clunie Press, 1987, 164–178.

Herzog, J. (1992). *L'insegnamento della lingua materna: aspetti del dialogo evolutivo figlia-padre*, In: Rosenfeld D. et al., *La funzione paterna*, Borla, Roma 1995, 15–38.

Holditch-Davis, D. et al. (1996). *Early parental interaction with and perceptions of multiple birth infants*, In: "Journal of Advanced Nursing", 30 (1), 200–210.

Hug-Hellmuth, H. (1921). *Vom mittleren Kind*, In "Imago", VII, 1921, pp. 179–197.

Isaacs, S. (1946). *Temper Tantrums in early childhood in their relation to internal objects in Childhood and After: some essays and clinical studies*, New York, International Universities Press Inc.

Jeammet, P. (1992). *La psicopatologia dell'adolescenza*, Roma, Borla.

Kancyper, L. (1997). *Il confronto generazionale. Uno studio psicoanalitico*, Milano, Franco Angeli, 2000.

Klein, M. (1932). *The Psychoanalysis of Children*. London, Hogarth Press.

Kris, M. & Ritvo, S. (1983). *Parents and siblings*, In: "The Psychoanalytic Study of the Child", 38, 311–324.

Laufer, M. & Laufer, E.M. (1984). *Adolescence and Developmental Breakdown: A Psychoanalytic View*, London, Karnac Books.

Lecourt, E. (2003). *La fraternalità del gemello. Il doppio, il gruppo, il collettivo*, In: M.L. Algini (Ed.), *Fratelli* cit., 172–184.

Leichtman, M. (1985). *The influence of an older sibling on the separation-individuation process*, In: "The Psychoanalytic Study of the Child", 40, 111–161.

Levi D'Ancona, V. et al. (1982). *The Florence sextuplets. Report of a case. Part one: Study of the patient, the onset of pregnancy and its early stages*, In: "Acta Europea Fertilitatis", vol. 13, n. 1, 19–23.

Lorenz, K. (1935). *Le compagnon dans l'environnement propre de l'oiseau*, In: *Essais sur le comportement animal et humain*, Paris, Seuil, 1970.

Magagna, J. et al. (2005). *Intimate Transformations*, London, Karnac.

Maiello, S. (1993). *L'oggetto sonoro. Un'ipotesi sulle radici prenatali della memoria uditiva*, In: "Richard & Piggle", vol. 1, n. 1, 31–47.

Meltzer, D. (1979). *Teoria psicoanalitica dell'adolescenza* In: "Quaderni di psicoterapia infantile", 1, Roma, Borla, 15–32.

Meltzer, D. (1984). *Dream-Life: a Re-examination of the Psycho-analytic Theory and Technique*, Perthshire, Clunie Press.

Meltzer, D. & Harris, M. (1983). *Child, Family and Community: a psycho-analytical model of the learning process*, Organisation for Economic Co-operation and Development, Paris.

Mitchell, J. (2000). *Mad Men and Medusa. Reclaiming Hysteria and the Effect of Sibling Relations in the Human Condition*. London, Penguin.

Mitchell, J. (2003). *I fratelli e la genesi del genere*, paper read at the Istituto Italiano per gli Studi Filosofici. Napoli. March 2003.

Moreno, J.L. (1964). *Principi di sociometria, di psicoterapia di gruppo e di sociodramma*, Milano. Etas Kompass.

Mori, L. (2004). *L'apporto dell'esperienza fraterna allo sviluppo psichico e alla costruzione dell'identità individuale*, In: "Contrappunto", 35, 35–60.

Negri, R. (1994). *Il neonato in terapia intensiva*. Milano. Cortina.

Neubauer, P.B. (1982). *Rivalry, envy and jealousy*. In: "The Psychoanalytic Study of the Child", 37, 121–142.

Palacio-Espasa, F. (1999). *La psicoterapia psicoanalitica del paziente borderline*, paper read at the Associazione Fiorentina di Psicoterapia Psicoanalitica. Firenze. October 1999.

Passi Tognazzo, D. (1975). *Metodi e tecniche nella diagnosi della personalità*. Firenze. Giunti Barbèra.

Passi Tognazzo, D. (1979). *Il metodo Rorschach*. Firenze. Giunti Barbèra.

Piontelli, A. (1992). *From Fetus to Child. An Observational and Psychoanalytic Study*, London and New York Tavistock/Routledge.

Rabain, J. (1985). *La rivalità fraterna* In: Lebovici S., Diatkine S, Soulé M. (Ed.), *Trattato di psichiatria dell'infanzia e dell'adolescenza*. Roma. Borla. 1990, 241–262.

Reyes De Polanco, N. (2002). *Un cuatrillizo compartiendo al objeto materno*, paper read at The VI International Conference on Infant Observation. Krakow. July 2002.

Reyes De Polanco, N. (2004). *From Absolute Dependence to Relative Dependence in Quadruplets*, paper read at The VII International Conference on Infant Observation. Firenze, April 2004.

Root Fortini, L. & Mori, L. (2002). *A retrospective study of sextuplets: Some predictive factors for personality development*, paper read at The VI International Conference on Infant Observation, Krakow, July 2002.

Root Fortini, L. & Mori, L. (2004). *From Pregnancy to Mothering Multiples*, paper read at The VII International Conference on Infant Observation. Firenze, April 2004.

Rosenfeld, D. (1992). *Il ruolo del padre nella psicosi*. In: Rosenfeld D. et al., *La funzione paterna*, Borla, Roma 1995, 15–38.

Schachter, F.F. (1976). *Sibling deidentification*, In: "Child Development Psychology", Barnard College 1976 (sept.), vol. XII (5), 418–427.

Schachter, & Frances Fuchs (1978). *Sibling deidentification judged by mothers: cross validation and developmental studies*, In: "Child Developments", 49.

Schowalter, & John, E. (1983). *Disturbi affettivi e malattie fisiche nell'infanzia*, In: H. Golombek e B.D. Garfinkel, *I disturbi affettivi dell'adolescenza*. Roma. Armando, 1990.

Sharpe, S.A. & Rosenblatt, A.D. (1994). *Oedipal sibling triangles*, In: "Journal of the American Psychoanalytic Association", 42, 491–523.

Soifer, R. (1985). *Psicodinamica della gravidanza, del parto e del puerperio,* Roma, Borla.

Stern, D.N. (1985). *The Interpersonal World of the Infant.* New York. Basic Books.

Sulloway, F.I. (1996). *Born to Rebel: Birth Order, Family Dynamics, and Creative Lives,* London, Abacus, 1998.

Suomi, S.J. (1982). *Sibling relatonships in nonhuman primates.* In: M.E. Lamb & B. Sutton-Smith, *Sibling relationships: their nature and significance across the life span,* New Jersey, Hillsdale, 329–356.

Taddei, I. (2000). *Relazioni fraterne. Uno sguardo sulla prima infanzia,* Gruppalità e Ciclo Vitale, Psychomedia Telematic Review.

Vallino, D. (1996). *Un quadro vivente dello sviluppo mentale nell'Infant Observation. Funzioni e disfunzioni dell'osservatore e del gruppo di dis-cussione,* In: "Quaderni di Psicoterapia Infantile", 33, 19–52.

Vallino, D. & Macciò, M. (2004). *Essere neonati. Questioni psiconalit-iche,* Roma, Borla.

Wallon, H. (1941). *Evolution Psychique de l'Enfant.* Paris. A. Colin.

Winnicott, D. (1935). *The manic defense,* In: *Collected Papers: Through Pediatrics to Psycho-Analysis.* London. Tavistock Publications, 1958.

Winnicott, D. (1945). *The only child,* In: *The Child, the Family and the Outside World.* London. Penguin Books, 1991, 131–136

Zazzo, R. (1960). *Les jumeaux, le couple et la personne.* Paris, Quadrige/Puf.

Zazzo, R. (1997). *Le paradoxe des jumeaux.* Paris. Editions Stock/ Laurence Pernoud.

# *INDEX*

Adler, Alfred 86
Alice 23
  at nursery school 44–45
  closing analysis 109
  drawing 102
  ego-synchronic way 45
  family drawing 101, 107–108
  first impressions 40–41
  firstborn 40
  internal organs drawing 108
  personality traits
    and relational
    characteristics 45–46
  play 42
  progress 41–42
  psycho-motor development 45
  relationship between the two
    sisters 43–44
  relationship with father 42
  socio-relational
    questionnaire 109–110

  special relationship with her
    father 45
  top student 96
  WAIS 109
  written self-presentation
    108–109
Alimentary idiosyncrasies 82
Animalism 74
Ascher, R.L. 104
Assistant for Affection 14
Authoritarian child 87

Background noise 16
Bettelheim 79
Bick, Esther 2, 61, 80
  method 3
Bisexual pubertal group
  mentality 112
Brotherly love 80
Brunet-Lezine test 3, 21, 39, 44, 124
Bruno 20–21

at nursery school 50–51
Brunet-Lezine test 50
closing analysis 112
family drawing 101, 110–111
first impressions 46–47
internal organs
    drawing 102, 111
Meltzer's description 112
motor difficulties 47–48
neuromotor-relational
    evaluation 46
personality traits and relational
    characteristics 51
play girl-type games 48
play 48–49
socio-relational questionnaire
    111–112
solitary child 46
temperamental
    behaviour 49–50
WAIS 111
written self-presentation 111

Carlo 21
Brunet-Lezine test 54–55
damaged child 51
family drawing 113
first impressions 51–53
internal organs
    drawing 102, 113
one-to-one relationship with an
    adult figure 55
overall analysis 114
personality traits and relational
    characteristics 55–56
problems 97
psycho-motor development 55
relationship with the other
    sextuplets 53
socio-relational
    questionnaire 113
temper tantrums 54

WAIS 113
written self-presentation 113
Case Western Research
    University 124
Chaos
    children were
        everywhere 75, 83
Child-parent relationships.,
Children's
    cushion effect 130
    different care taking styles 25
    11th observation 27
    leave-taking 35–36
    lunchtime 22
    neuro-psychiatrist 39
    objective proof of
        differences 21–22
    observation at the nursery
        school 32
    psychic health 18
    psycho-motor development 22
    scenes from everyday life 22–25
    second year, "the children are
        everywhere" 28
    7th observation 23–25
    10th observation 26
    third year, "staying at home is
        a disaster" 36–38
    12th observation 27
    20th observation 24–25
Coles, P. 79–80, 127
Commanding and intrusive 97
Comparetti, Adriano Milani 39

Daniele 21, 23
    at nursery school 60
    Brunet-Lezine test 60
    community service work 95
    daring 58–59
    family drawing 114
    first impressions 56–57
    forgotten child 56

hyperactivity 57–58
internal organs
    drawing 102, 115
misunderstandings 59–60
needs and behavior 59
neuromotor-relational
    evaluation 56
overall analysis 116
personality traits
    and relational
    characteristics 61
problem 126
socio-relational
    questionnaire 115
WAIS 115
written self-presentation 115
Dann, Sophie 45
Darwinian principle 86
De-twinning or de-tripleting 81
Diversity 85
Donzelli, Giampaolo 3
Dunn, J. 114

Egocentric attitude 96
Ego-synchronic way 45
Elisa 23
    at nursery school 65
    Brunet-Lezine test 64–65
    conflicts and contrasts 63–64
    excellent achievement 119
    family drawing 117–119
    first impressions 61–62
    grandma's "pet" 61
    internal organs
        drawing 102, 117
    neuromotor-relational
        evaluation 61
    Oedipal triangles 64
    overall analysis 118–119
    personality traits
        and relational
        characteristics 65–66

sociability 62–63
socio-relational
    questionnaire 118
WAIS 118
written self-presentation
    117–118
Exclusive relationships
    one-to-one contact with the
        mother 85

Family-couple 15
Father-daughter relationship 91
Female band 15
Filippini, Filippo 4, 99
First birthday 17–18
First differences 15–17
First observation,
    "now we are ten" 11–13
Firstborns 88, 108, 126
Follow-up visits and
    psychological tests 94
    first 94–96
    second 96–98
    third 98–99
Fortini, Linda Root 3, 104
Franco 20–21, 23
    at nursery school 71
    baby boy 66
    Brunet-Lezine test 71
    family drawing 101, 119–120
    first impressions 66–67
    internal organs drawing 119
    Meltzer's description 121
    neuromotor-relational
        evaluation 66
    overall analysis 121
    personality traits and relational
        characteristics 71–72
    play 69–71
    relationship with the
        mother 67–68
    sociability 68–69

socio-relational
   questionnaire 120–121
WAIS 120
written self-presentation 120
Freud, Anna 45

Gazzarini, Edda 3
Gonadotropins 8
Going home 10–11

Hack, Maureen 124
Harris, M. 78
Heterosexual adolescents 112
Homogeneous group
   being part of 75–81
   sextuplet's experience 75
Homogeneous nestling-group 82
Hormone treatment 8, 73

Infancy and childhood
   seen through infant
   observation 7–38
   being in six 73–92
   closing comments 129–132
   different care taking
     styles 25–28
   11th observation 27
   father 18–21
   follow-up fifteen years
     later 93–127
   first birthday 17–18
   first differences 15–17
   first observation,
     "now we are ten" 11–13
   4th observation 23
   going home 10–11
   individual evaluations 107–127
   leave-taking 35–36
   neuromotor-relational
     examination 90
   objective proof of
     differences 21–22

observation at nursery
   school 32–34
organization of an enlarged
   family 13–15
pregnancy and birth 8–10
scenes from everyday life 22
second year 28–32
7th observation 23–25
10th observation 26
third year, "staying at home is
   a disaster" 36–38
three follow-up home visits
   93–94
12th observation 27–28
20th observation 24–25
*Infant Observation* 1–2
   groups 3
   method 5
   stages 2
   infancy and childhood 7–38
Inside-of-the-Body-Test 104
Intra-uterine space 84

Klein, M. 78
Kyrle, Money 126

Life events
   in late adolescence 123

Maternal identity, atypical 73–75
Maternal service 14
Mazzetti, Daisy 3
Meltzer's description 112, 121
Mori, Gina Ferrara 2–3
Mori, Laura 4, 105
MOST (mothers of
   super twins) 124
Mother-baby-sextuplet group
   relationships 2
Mother-child
   couple 78
   relationship 2, 79, 130–131

Mother-child-sextuplet group
    relationship 81–85
Mother-daughter
    identification 110
    conflict 110
Mother hen 98
Mother's
    ambivalent feelings 27
    exceptional pregnancy 110
    manic self-defence 75
    preoccupations 96
Mother unconscious feelings 88
Motor difficulties 47–48
Movie star 14
Mummy's sweeties 25

Neuromotor-relational
    evaluation 40
    examination 90
*New England Journal of Medicine* 124
Nicoletti, Ivan 3
Non-antagonistic parental
    couple 15
Non-incestuous love 80

Oedipal
    desire 117
    drama 80
    parental triangles 89
    rivalry 45
    sibling triangle 117
    triangles 64
One-to-one relationships 91
One-to-two parent-children
    ratio 113
Organization of an enlarged
    family 13–15

Palacio-Espasa 61
Personality tests, projective 99–104
Piontelli's
    longitudinal observational 76

Pregnancy and birth 8
Pre-oedipal phase 89
Pre-school age siblings 78
Primordial fear 110
Protagonist 10
Psycho-affective development 131
Psycho-cognitive development 4
Psycho-diagnostic tests 99–107
Psychodynamic profiles
    of individual sextuplets 39–72
Psycho-motor development
    45, 55, 124
Psychophysical development 87
Psycho-sexual
    identity 121–122, 126
    in adolescence 103
Public domain 14

Relational model 82
Ruocco, Mario 4, 104

Sextuplets
    affective-relational life of 76
    continuity and discontinuity in
        development 122
    "cushion effect" on personality
        development 80
    development and important
        events 93
    essential data 40
    individual 4
    maternal grandparents 8
    psychodynamic profiles 39–72
    research methods and
        structure 1–5
    sibling group 127
Sforza, Angela 4, 104
Sharing
    each child had one-sixth of the
        mother 84
Sibling
    experience 80

relationships 1, 77, 80
    understanding 92
Sibling rivalry 78
Socio-relational
    development 99
Socio-relational questionnaire 93,
    97, 104–107, 125
    relationships with brothers
        and sisters 106
Start-and-stop relationships 83
"Super" father 89
"Super" mother 89, 99

Tactile-auditory sensations 76
Tait, C.B. 104
Temper tantrums 54
Temperamental behaviour 49–50
Theresienstadt concentration
    camp 45

Tognazzo, Passi 103, 117, 119, 121
Tranquillizing warmth 76
Triplets-quadruplets-
    quintuplets-sextuplets 81
Twins-triplets 81

Unconscious Labels 81
Unconscious parental
    attitudes 81

Vecchi, Corrado 3

WAIS 4, 95, 104, 109, 111,
    113–114
Winnicott
    BBC radio interview 19

Yale University Study Group 78
Young parental couple 15